Rolling
WORKOUT

**THE REVOLUTIONARY WAY
TO TONE, LENGTHEN, AND
REALIGN YOUR BODY**

Yamuna Zake and Stephanie Golden

Broadway Books
New York

BROADWAY

PRINTED IN THE UNITED STATES OF AMERICA

BROADWAY BOOKS and its logo, a letter B bisected on the diagonal, are trademarks of Random House, Inc.

Visit our website at www.broadwaybooks.com

First edition published 2003.

Book design by Lee Fukui

Library of Congress Cataloging-in-Publication Data
Zake, Yamuna, 1954–
    The Ultimate body rolling workout : the revolutionary way to tone, lengthen, and
  realign your body / Yamuna Zake, with Stephanie Golden.
      p. cm.
    1. Massage. 2. Exercise. 3. Physical fitness. I. Golden, Stephanie. II. Title.
RM721.Z247 2003
613.7'1—dc22
                                                                                2003058530

ISBN 0-7679-1230-6

10 9 8 7 6 5

The ULTIMATE
Body Rolling
WORKOUT

The ULTIMATE
Body

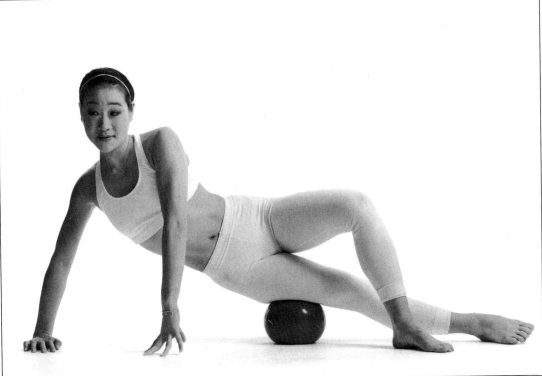

Contents

Acknowledgments

First of all I thank my parents, who opened their home to Stephanie Golden and to me, providing us with a beautiful place to do the major conceptual work on this book.

I thank Stephanie for being so incredibly amazing to work with. I feel blessed to have found a writer who is so professional, believes totally in the work, and understands what I want to say.

Many thanks to Mitchell Waters, my agent at Curtis Brown, and his assistant, Kirsten Manges, who believed right away that Body Rolling could be the next big thing in fitness.

Special thanks to Ann Campbell, my editor at Broadway, who recognized this book as the initiator of a new, important, and powerful body of work combining fitness, massage, and healing; and to her assistant, Jenny Cookson, for helping with all the minutiae that go into producing a really complicated book.

Tim Geaney's wonderfully upbeat nature, plus his ability to take just the right shot, made the photos for this book beautiful as well as informative.

I thank Ivanna Wei, Daniella Ubide, and my daughter, Yael Zake Becker, for modeling the routines.

I am deeply grateful to my husband, Jonathan Paskow, for his integral help with all the business aspects of my work and especially for his love and support and his understanding of the amount of time that goes into creating a book.

The certified Body Rolling practitioners were the first people to recognize the potential of Body Rolling. From their own experience of this work, they knew it would have a strong impact in the world of health and fitness and wanted to be part of it from the very beginning. I am thankful for their continuing support.

Finally, I thank all my clients, who have always been my teachers. From them I've learned everything I know about the body. Now, with Body Rolling, they have a tool to learn about and heal their own bodies.

I dedicate this book to my father, Lawrence Zake, who was always my biggest fan. He believed in my work from the beginning, supported me, and encouraged me. From him I drew the courage to keep on, no matter how much my work ran counter to conventional beliefs about fitness and about the body.

1

Roll Your Way to a Better Body

Wouldn't you like your body to look and function better, *without* all the work that most fitness programs require? Body Rolling, an exercise program that you do with a ball, will tone, strengthen, and realign your body in a way that's not only easy but enjoyable and extraordinarily effective. This cutting-edge fitness practice—which isn't just for fitness buffs—will make you leaner, longer, and stronger; you'll achieve a terrific shape that you can't get from other workouts. Body Rolling will also prevent and fix all sorts of body problems. It's a workout, a massage, and a chiropractic session all in one!

What makes Body Rolling special is that you achieve phenomenal results in your very first session. Immediately, your whole body feels transformed: you're breathing more deeply; you're standing differently on your legs; your joints are looser. When you look in the mirror, you see clear, obvious changes: you're taller; your posture is better; you look sleeker, longer, and more shaped. And you suddenly feel an amazing sense of ease and well-being throughout your body.

From the start, Body Rolling goes to work on precisely those parts of your physique that are key to your particular self-image and sense of well-being. Laura, for example, had always felt bottom-heavy. She tried the treadmill, running, and stretching, but nothing succeeded in toning and slimming her heavy hips and thighs. So in her first Body Rolling class, she did the routines for the legs, rolling the ball down the front, back, inside, and outside of both thighs. When she finished and stood up, she exclaimed, "Oh, my god—my legs feel longer! I'm standing differently. I feel taller, and I'm even walking more easily. It's hard to believe this, but I also feel thinner! I can hardly believe I got this many changes from one session of just rolling on a ball!"

When Laura actually looked in the mirror, she saw that not only was she standing taller, but her legs were visibly thinner, toned, and more shaped. After spending so many weeks in the gym working intensely to slim her thighs, she couldn't understand how something as simple as Body Rolling could create such big changes so fast—but she was thrilled.

After class, Jackie listened to Laura describe these astonishing results while absently zipping up her skirt. Suddenly she stopped and stared at her waistline. "Oh, wow—my skirt is big on me! Can you believe it? How did this happen in a single class?" For Jackie the key Body Rolling routines were the ones for the back and front of her torso. These routines stretched out all her abdominal muscles and the long muscles running up her back—which meant that, like Laura, she was now taller. As those muscles elongated, they grew narrower, hence her smaller waist.

Laura and Jackie aren't unusual. *Everyone* feels major changes after their first Body Rolling session. Suddenly they're standing more upright, with their shoulders dropped back and down, and their neck longer and moving more easily. They find they no longer have to *work* at standing straight or trying to hold their abdomen in or preventing their shoulders from rounding forward. This is because all the Body Rolling routines build core strength, which is what you need to stand up tall.

Body Rolling realigns your body, bringing all the parts back to where they're supposed to be. You start feeling "right" in your body. Some people even remark that they never dreamed they could feel so peaceful and comfortable in their bodies, so much calmer and more relaxed. And they realize that whatever has happened goes beyond just working their muscles, for standing taller makes them feel better about themselves overall. The powerful awareness that your body has just gone through a major transformative change is one of the great gifts of Body Rolling.

Another stand-out benefit is that just by doing the basic routines in this book, you'll be able to prevent common discomforts such as tension, tightness, and pain. And if you already have a problem that's bothering you, Body Rolling will start to relieve it. This also means that you can avoid the stiffness, loss of mobility, and other problems that most people accept as natural when they get older. With Body Rolling you never have to grow stiff and weak; you can live out your later years with remarkable strength and vitality.

What Is Body Rolling?

Body Rolling evolved out of Body Logic, a body therapy I developed about twenty years ago, which is based on the principle that most people suffer pain and restricted movement due to faulty body alignment that results in collapsed posture, muscle tightness, and pressure on nerves. In treating people with Body Logic, I exerted traction on muscle by using one elbow to put pressure where a muscle began and the other hand to pull the muscle in the direction of its natural movement. Once it was elongated, the muscle could take up its full length, decompressing bones, joints, and nerves and restoring full function.

After practicing Body Logic and training other practitioners to do it in New York for several years, I moved to Spain, where I had no one who could work on me. So I decided to invent a way in which a ball could act as a practitioner's hands and proceeded to translate Body Logic onto the ball.

The result was Body Rolling, which consists of a series of routines that use a six- to ten-inch-diameter inflatable ball to stretch muscles, freeing restrictions in all parts of the body, increasing blood flow, and promoting healing. Lying over the ball, you literally roll your body out almost like dough, stretching and elongating your muscles. The Body Rolling routines follow specific sequences that match the body's own logic and order. Starting where each muscle begins, at the point called its origin, you roll toward its insertion, the point where it attaches to the bone that it moves. Unlike other types of ball work, Body Rolling allows you to work specific muscles in detail. You can even get into tight, restricted areas and loosen the muscles up.

Many people now use balls of different sizes for stretching, physical therapy, core strengthening, and balance. These programs consist of individual exercises targeted to specific body parts. But Body Rolling is different, for it stretches, tones, and realigns your whole body, as well as developing core strength. I think of Body Rolling more as a lifestyle than just a fitness program, since when you're more at ease in your body, your whole life feels easier.

No matter who you are, Body Rolling should be part of your life. And making it an everyday habit is easy, because you can do it at home, as part of your workout, or at the office. I've created office routines that prevent headaches; back, neck, and shoulder tension; and repetitive syndromes such as carpal tunnel that result from hours sitting at a desk or computer. You can also deflate the ball and take it on the road. Travelers find that using Body Rolling on airplanes and in hotels prevents jet lag and improves their performance, since their bodies aren't sluggish and aching. And, since most people have a limited amount of time, I've created routines you can do in just a few minutes for specific parts of the body: rolling up the spine, for example, is a great way to relax before going to sleep or to relieve the stiffness many people feel upon waking.

Everyone Benefits

I've never known a single person who hasn't seen amazing results from Body Rolling. Whether you're young and fit and feeling on top of the world or older and more seasoned, you'll see dramatic improvements. You might not yet realize what "better" can be for you, but Body Rolling will reveal your own version of it.

DEDICATED ATHLETES

People who are serious about their workouts, such as athletes and dancers, seek peak performance; Body Rolling can help them achieve this. For example, a runner who wants to speed up his time can use the ball to work all his thigh muscles. As he does the routines, he begins to sense which of those muscles are tight and restricting his movement. At the same time, the routines release those muscles, so he moves more freely when he runs and his time improves. Golfers can work out their back twist and prevent lower back problems. And Body Rolling will directly improve their swing.

In many ways, Body Rolling is the perfect manifestation of the new mind-body trend in fitness, as well as the current shift away from earlier motivating concepts like "no pain, no gain" for athletes. In more than twenty years as a body therapist, I've found that many people who go to great lengths to be fit—running, working out at gyms, learning Pilates, practicing yoga—often wind up hurting themselves by doing repetitive movements with bodies that aren't properly aligned. Many others walk around with pain and restrictions that they're only half aware of and accept as inevitable, because they don't know how easily these problems can be fixed. Because Body Rolling automatically restores your body to its correct alignment, it prepares you to do any type of exercise without injury, and it helps muscle tears heal faster.

While Body Rolling is an essential complement to any fitness program, on its own it provides many of the benefits of popular workout systems like Gyrotonics and Pilates, at far less expense. It requires only a ball and a book or video, and it can be practiced at home.

Couch Potatoes

Many people aren't interested in working out. They basically feel fine in their bodies and just want to stay reasonably in shape. To them, the feeling of "better" after a Body Rolling session comes as a surprise, for they hadn't realized how much of an improvement in their physical well-being was actually possible. For these people, as well as those who don't really enjoy exercise but feel they ought to do it—or are told by a doctor that they must—Body Rolling offers an experience that's inviting, instead of being a chore. You don't have to work hard to achieve a toned, well-aligned body—and it's fun! Some people don't particularly like going to the gym; they have to force themselves to work out. But Body Rolling is so easy, and feels so good, that even non-exercisers get hooked. And because they see truly fantastic results quickly, they stick with the program. The more they do it, the greater their results.

A Simple Way to Slim Down

Many overweight people feel uncomfortable and unwelcome at gyms, making exercise even more of an obstacle. Yet these people too will find Body Rolling not only doable but enjoyable. After their first session, overweight people usually feel uplifted. Their weight pulls their body down but right away Body Rolling begins to reverse that, so they feel taller and freer in their movement. This gives them an incentive to do more. And because Body Rolling stimulates the nerve roots (which emerge from the spinal cord to form the major sensory and motor nerves, each innervating a different part of the body), it also stimulates the vital organs, improves circulation, and boosts metabolism, so all the body systems begin to function better. In this way, Body Rolling can actually help them lose weight.

Often people try to shed pounds by doing cardiovascular workouts to burn calories. Or they try weight training, hoping they'll lose weight as well as build healthy muscle mass. They're afraid that if they don't burn enough calories, they'll put on pounds. Yet often a rigorous workout will increase your appetite. But because Body Rolling relaxes you instead of depleting you, your need to eat actually decreases.

An Amazing New Look

As Laura's and Jackie's experiences show, Body Rolling also changes your appearance in ways you will love. Often people tell me that their friends ask, "What are you doing? You look thinner." In fact, they aren't thinner, but their whole body is longer, so they appear thinner. As Jackie discovered, elongating the muscles of your back, sides, and abdomen lengthens your torso and flattens your stomach. Most people find themselves tightening their belts another notch, and their clothes feel looser. Some women go down a whole dress size. The Body Rolling leg and pelvis routines perk up sagging buttocks, and the ball breaks up fatty deposits (otherwise known as cellulite), which is another reason that your thighs will start looking more streamlined.

Wrinkles on the face, sagging cheeks, double chins, and lines in the neck all result from your head dropping down into your neck, so that the muscles of your face collapse. When you elongate and tone the neck muscles, they hold the head up properly, so the sagging skin under your neck disappears and your wrinkles smooth out.

Beat the Clock and Age Gracefully

Picture two women walking down the street. One takes elastic strides, head erect, arms swinging freely. The other woman's head sinks forward, her spine slumps, her shoulders round, her chest is concave, her belly protrudes and sags. Because this posture limits her movement, she walks with a shuffle. From a distance, this second woman appears much older. But they're actually both twenty-eight.

Despite her youth, the second woman has fallen into the classic aging posture. No matter how old you are chronologically, this pose ages you. It doesn't just make you *look* older; it promotes structural and physiological aging processes in your body. And it can begin at any time, whatever your size, shape, or ethnic and racial background may be. Sooner or later, most people wind up in this posture—simply because they have never paid attention to how they were using their bodies. They look old at way too young an age.

Many people, particularly women, think of wrinkles as the ultimate harbinger of age. In fact, it's bad posture that causes wrinkles. Your skin is the clothing for your muscles, so if your muscles aren't toned, your skin will sag. My mother used to say that you can always tell a woman's age by her neck. And certainly, if you're frozen into the aging posture, your neck sags along with everything else. But if you remain upright, your neck muscles work properly and remain long. They stretch the skin out, and it doesn't droop.

What really determines how young you look and feel is how freely you move. Cosmetic surgery may change your appearance, but it can't make you feel or even look young if your body can't move. Once you've assumed the aging posture, your bones harden into position and restrict muscle movement, so the muscles in turn lose their range of motion. Eventually the posture restricts shoulder and leg movements, limits breathing capacity, and causes neck and lower back pain. The abdomen drops forward and weakens the abdominal muscles, so the intestines slip downward, exerting pressure on the pelvis.

Ultimately the posture leads to height loss, arthritis, and osteoporosis.

But *this aging process of stiffness and contraction doesn't have to happen.* Recent research shows that you don't have to lose muscle quality as you grow older; you can build muscle mass and increase strength at any age. Body Rolling offers a fast, easy way to improve your posture now and keep your muscles elongated, flexible, and toned, so you don't get old and stiff while you're still young—or ever.

Of all the preventive strategies available today to help people look better and stay healthier and more active, Body Rolling is one of the best, for it keeps you young by keeping your bones and muscles healthy—free to move easily your entire life. Even if you've already noticed some restrictions, it's never too late to regain the range of movement you've lost.

A New Perspective on Osteoporosis

These days, the brittle bones of osteoporosis are a widespread fear for women, beginning as early as the late twenties for some. Many come to me in a panic after bone scans showing that their bone density is way down. They're terrified to do anything with their bodies, even the fitness practices they've already been doing. But I explain that this diagnosis doesn't mean they're suddenly going to crack apart. They can still continue with the exercise their body is used to—although this isn't the time to start some new high-impact routine. Rather, it's a time to take steps to improve bone quality. Instead of using the term *osteoporosis,* I tell them, think about it as bone that is challenged and needs extra help. Just as you work muscle to improve its quality, you can also work bone.

In starting a program to improve your bone quality, it's important to understand that bone is living tissue. As in every part of the body, age brings wear and tear to bone. Years of pounding from running, for example, cause microtrauma that cut off circulation. The bone becomes brittle and its supply of nutrients is diminished. To me, brittle bone is like dried fruit. Just as a raisin plumps up when you put it in water, when you directly stimulate bone it undergoes a similar change and becomes more flexible.

Weight-bearing exercise helps build bone density by providing just such stimulation. Research has shown that as muscles and tendons contract during weight-bearing exercise and hit against the bone, they stimulate the cells that create bone tissue. Many varieties of weight-bearing exercise are available, including yoga, Pilates, and weight lifting. I see many people who hear that weight-bearing exercise is important, so they run out and do whatever form of it the magazines say is the hot new trend. Yet if their alignment is poor, they may wind up injuring their joints. So I recommend that whichever form of exercise you choose, take the time to do Body Rolling first, to align the joints you want to strengthen.

And if weight-bearing exercise doesn't appeal to you, Body Rolling all by itself is also an excellent way to improve bone quality. It's actually a mild form of weight-bearing exercise, in which the weight of your body sinking into the ball applies pressure directly into the bone to stimulate the bone-building cells—more directly even than lifting weights. The pressure brings increased circulation to bone, tendons, and muscles, all at the same time. One woman whose osteoporosis was documented by a bone scan showed a significant improvement in bone density after a year of practicing Body Rolling. Another woman, in her late fifties, grew one-third of an inch taller after six months of practice.

What's more, Body Rolling is safe, since as you do it you're correcting your alignment and increasing your flexibility and muscle tone. As a bonus, keeping your body flexible means you'll be less likely to break a bone should you fall. If you do have osteoporosis or any other kind of bone abnormality, show your doctor these routines and get his or her approval before beginning Body Rolling. Finally, *be sure that you use a soft ball* (see pages 42–43).

More pleasurable lovemaking: Lovemaking is a physical activity, and the freer and more flexible your pelvis, the more intense your sexual response. If you're stiff and restricted, fewer positions are available to you. Body Rolling begins immediately to free your pelvis, so you can loosen up and let go.

A stronger voice: Singers tell me that Body Rolling frees their throat, opens their chest, and increases lung capacity, so their voice grows stronger.

Relief from pain: One of my clients, a man with crippling sciatica, slept pain-free for the first time in two years after just one Body Rolling session.

Feel better when you're pregnant: If you're pregnant, the Body Rolling back, side, and leg routines will keep your posture straight, ward off lower back pain, and create more abdominal space for the baby to grow in.

Emotional release: Body Rolling brings emotional as well as physical benefits. You can roll away everyday stress, anxiety, irritation, or pent-up anger, keeping yourself on a more even keel. After a difficult day, a few minutes of Body Rolling can make you feel peaceful again. People even use it as a form of meditation to calm and soothe mind and body.

Feel It, Find It, and Fix It Yourself!

Of all the benefits of Body Rolling, the most important is this: you can use it to learn what's going on in your own body. You can discover and fix potential problems at an early stage, before they get so bad you need to see a doctor or body therapist.

Kathy had no problems in her body that she knew of, though she was vaguely aware that her right side felt a bit tighter than the left.

When she got up from her chair after hours of leaning over her desk, for example, she sensed some tightness in her right hip. But when she tried Body Rolling and rolled the ball down the backs of her legs, she had a clear, specific sensation of exactly how much tighter her right leg was than the left one. When she stood up after finishing the leg routine, her whole right side, and especially the connection between her right hip and leg, felt looser and freer.

Next Kathy did the back routine and noticed that it was easier to roll up the left side of her back than the right side. On the left side, she could feel her spine lengthening and her muscles releasing as the ball moved upward. But on the right, it was harder to get that feeling. This told her that the whole right side of her back, too, was more contracted than the left side—something she hadn't been aware of. Then, when she stood up, she could feel that the two sides had become equally elongated: her whole spine felt taller. In this way Kathy discovered her own level of "better" that she hadn't dreamed existed. But what most amazed her were the changes in the rest of her body. Not only was her back longer, but her arms no longer rotated forward, and her neck didn't thrust her head in front of her.

All these discoveries set Kathy's mind working. "Why was I so much tighter on the right?" she wondered. "What do I do differently on that side?" She had to think for only a minute or two before she realized that as she sat at her desk all day, she was putting more pressure on her right side: sitting more heavily on her right buttock and leaning to the right as she wrote with her right hand.

Body Rolling can also help you find solutions to problems you may have had for a long time, as you begin to learn what I call the *language of the body*: the sensations that tell you what's going on inside your body. When your body presses into the ball, you feel a specific sensation that your mind then registers—just as Kathy felt that her right leg muscles were tighter than those on the left. This is the Body Rolling *body-mind dialogue*, and it can be tremendously revealing (see pages 34–36).

Suppose you're aware at the end of the day that your neck and shoulders feel tight because you slouch a bit while you work. Maybe you've tried to work out that tension or had someone rub your shoulders, but you didn't get any results. But when you try the Body Rolling neck and shoulder routines, that tension just disappears. Since you love the feeling of being without it, you continue using Body Rolling every day to roll the tension out of your muscles.

Whether it's your neck or your hips or your back that's speaking to you, you'll find help in this book. Chapters 4 to 9 offer specific routines for different parts of the body, so you can choose the ones your body needs. You'll discover that the more you work on yourself—as opposed to having someone else do it for you—the more acute your body awareness will become. Body Rolling makes taking care of your body easy, especially since your body starts to love Body Rolling and practically insists that you get on the ball. Once you realign the parts that were slightly askew without your even being aware of it, you'll experience that wonderful sensation of "better."

How Body Rolling Works

The basic principle of Body Rolling is creating space. Just as people exclaim, "I need my own space!" every part of your body needs its proper space to function at its best. Pain or discomfort due to a sprain, muscle spasm, or pressure on a nerve is the result of compression—meaning lack of space—in the painful area. Lack of space first manifests as muscle tightness (you can't turn or bend as much as you could before). If you don't release this tightness, the muscles can become so tight that they press on a nerve, causing sciatica or numbness in your fingers or toes. And when muscles are contracted, the internal organs also have less space and receive less blood circulation, so their function slows.

Different bodies lack space for different reasons. Almost everyone has some muscles in their body that they don't use, and those areas have collapsed because the underused muscles have lost their ability to function properly. A muscle that stops functioning atrophies (that is, it starts to shrink and sag) and shortens, so it's no longer taking up its full space. Everyone's body also has areas where the muscles are overworked from holding the body in a particular posture. In this case the lack of space results from the tightness of these constantly contracted muscles.

Dedicated exercisers lack space for other reasons. Weight lifters working to bulk up their muscles, for example, often focus only on the central part of the muscle, because it's the part they can see. Instead of consciously working the whole muscle, they leave out the tendons (the two ends of the muscle that attach it to bone). As they keep bulking the muscle, it shortens, putting stress on the tendons. That's why most sports injuries are tendon strains. Shorter muscles also make joints tighter because they pull the bones together.

Body Rolling creates space in the body by elongating muscle. Once the muscles have their full length, they stop pressing into and irritating nerves, and the joints have space to move more freely. When you place the ball at the muscle's starting point, or origin, and allow your body weight to sink into it, you stimulate the tendon, which becomes more elastic, triggering a release through the entire muscle. As you roll toward the muscle's end point, or insertion, you deepen the release. Working with the ball reveals to you how tightness in certain muscles prevents certain joints from moving easily. As you start to release the muscles, the joint automatically loosens up.

Suppose that, like Kathy, you've noticed that your right leg doesn't move as freely from the hip as the left leg, so you use the ball to release your hamstrings (the back-of-thigh muscles). Now the leg feels freer, but it's still not walking as freely as the other leg. Next you work on the quadriceps (the front-of-thigh muscles), and the leg becomes freer still. Last, you roll out the adductors (the inner-thigh muscles) and find that the entire hip is moving freely. The message here is that your hip tightness resulted from contractions in three different muscle groups that all connect to the hip joint. Using the same kind of logical process in other parts of your body as you work with the ball, you begin to see how groups of muscles can be related to tightness in any area.

Ironing Out Your Muscles

Each type of tissue in our body—skin, muscle, fat, and bone—has its own purpose and needs to be separate from the other tissues in order to function optimally. But we all have particular habitual postures we fall into every day that cause these different tissues to get stuck to each other by connective tissue that glues them together. Over time, circulation decreases in these stuck areas, the skin sags, and fatty deposits (cellulite) accumulate.

We all have stuck places in our body—no matter how much of an athlete we may be, or how conscious of our body we think we are. And exercise by itself isn't enough to change the quality of this tissue; often the repetitive stress of exercise causes the tissues to stick together even more tightly. What Body Rolling does is unstick and decongest these tissues by literally ironing them out. The shapes of individual muscles begin to emerge out of what looked like a single mass, and wrinkles and sagging skin fill out.

Just Let Go!

We spend a great deal of time gripping: holding our body in some particular posture we assume to perform a certain practice. The classic example in everyday life is your parents reminding you, "Stand up straight!" Children try to oblige by holding their shoulders up in a forced position. By the time they're twenty, this tension pattern is ingrained in their bodies, and they maintain it the rest of their life. Many physical disciplines have a similar effect. A ballerina's body holds her training outside the dance studio, so she walks duck-footed.

A swimmer who does the crawl has shoulders that are raised and locked forward.

Unlike other exercise and body-therapy systems, Body Rolling's entire focus is on *letting go* of all that: both the patterns you've deliberately trained your body to hold and the ones you're completely unaware of. Generally, except in conscious relaxation or meditation practices, we don't embrace the concept of letting the body go; rather, we work to hold it or make it perform. What makes the Body Rolling transformation possible is that instead of holding your body in a certain way to perform a particular action, you release it.

Bob was a passionate golfer who worked with an instructor to improve his swing and the way he used his body. He took in the instructions mentally, working hard to get his positions perfect. Yet even as his mind commanded, "Stand like this, keep your hips like this, hold the club this way," tension built up in his body that continued to restrict his swing.

Hoping to increase his flexibility, Bob tried Body Rolling. After rolling up each side of his spine he immediately felt taller and freer, with a greater range of motion in his torso. The big change, however, occurred when he rolled up his chest and out to each shoulder. Even though the golf pro had said he needed ease in his arm movement, Bob hadn't realized how much tension he held in his shoulder in his effort to hold the club just right. When he stood up after doing the Body Rolling chest routine, Bob discovered that his arm movement was much freer. Then the next day, when he went out onto the course, he found himself actually experiencing the ease that the pro had been trying to teach him. The Body Rolling had liberated his body from a pattern he was mentally imposing on it, so the swinging movement came naturally and easily. For Bob this experience turned out to be a deep psychological release as well, for he realized that to free his body, he had to let go of his mind's effort at control, based on its concept of what his body *should* do.

Redefining Fitness

Body Rolling introduces a new concept of fitness: that *everybody* can be fit. As it stands, people have wildly varying ideas of what fitness is. For a man, it might be looking youthful and having muscle definition or being able to press 250 pounds. For a woman, it's often being sexy—which means, according to the reigning image today, thin, tight, hard, and toned. This notion of fitness usually involves losing inches and body fat so she can wear a size 4 instead of an 8.

When people have an *idea* of fitness like this stuck in their minds, they're likely to sabotage *true* fitness. One of my clients thought fitness meant cardiovascular capacity. He insisted on going to the gym and using the treadmill even though this exacerbated the effects of a lower back injury. To a young female client, fitness was being flexible, long, strong, and relaxed, so she turned to yoga. But yoga class only worsened the back pain she had started out with, and on top of that she developed pelvic pain. Believing that in the name of being fit, she had to "work through the pain," she wound up injuring herself. Not surprisingly, instead of helping her relax, the classes only made her more tense.

A popular concept today is core fitness, which involves strengthening the deep muscles of the lower torso. One of my clients decided he needed to develop core strength in order to relieve his lower back pain. So he turned to Pilates, a core fitness method. But as it happened, his hips were uneven; one was rotated forward, the other backward. Doing Pilates leg lifts with these hips—whose imbalance was the source of his pain in the first place—exacerbated his lower back problem: his pelvis was contracted so tightly that when he raised his leg, the whole pelvis followed. He couldn't keep both hips on the ground, where they were supposed to remain during the exercise. The twisting of the hips as the legs moved strained the lower back muscles. But if he had done Body Rolling before his Pilates workout, he would have corrected his hip alignment and could have done the leg lifts without hurting his back.

As these examples show, people often assume that "fitness" means cardiovascular capacity, muscle strength, stretching, and flexibility. These are all important qualities that everyone needs to some degree—but they're only *components* of fitness. They don't necessarily define what it means to be a fit person. Fitness is really a whole-being concept that takes your entire body structure into account. It can't be reduced to the components of exercise or certain styles of exercise. Physical exercise has become a science; it can be studied and measured. But fitness is a state of being that isn't definable by numbers; rather, it's different for everyone. Because current fitness myths imply that fitness is only achievable by athletes, non-exercisers assume they can't ever be fit. But this book will teach you to use Body Rolling to achieve your version of fitness, whether you exercise or not.

In my definition, fitness simply means that your body doesn't hold you back from doing what *you* want to do. You can be fit without going to the gym or being an exercise fanatic, since what your fitness is depends on what your needs are. With Body Rolling, you can maintain your body's capacity to function the way you need to for your particular lifestyle.

Body Rolling is a complete system of fitness because, recognizing that all the parts of you are connected, it works your whole body at once. You can get fit by doing just Body Rolling, or you can use Body Rolling to do any other fitness practice with a sensitive, alert whole-body awareness that will not only make your other practice more effective but also prevent any injury. Without sweating and burning, you can have the body you need—a body that enables you to do whatever you want and never quits on you. Fitness is *not* about pushing yourself. It doesn't have to be hard—and it doesn't have to hurt.

If You Exercise Regularly

In the past twenty years, we've learned a lot about the importance of staying in shape and how to care for our bodies. But fitness—and especially fitness for women—is a relatively new field, and we don't yet have all the information we need. The results of new, sophisticated studies of the effects of different fitness activities are only just coming in. Each year we discover that some types of fitness practices can actually be harmful. Running, for example, was widely promoted from the seventies to the nineties, but we're now getting results showing that long-term running can seriously injure the knees, ankles, hips, and spine. As our information improves, we must change certain concepts we believed in the past.

With people flocking to newly popular fitness disciplines, we must all remember that it takes years to acquire enough information to really understand their harms and benefits. This is why it's so important for everyone to learn to listen to their bodies, not just get stuck on an idea like "Running is good for me." Every exercise system has a possible downside. But with Body Rolling, you can have that workout you love and still avoid injury.

Fitness buffs can use Body Rolling as a prelude and/or finish to their workout. Doing it before your workout will warm up your muscles and increase range of motion, improving your performance. If you're doing really intense training, rolling your muscles out afterward will prevent tightness. There's no rule for when it's best to do Body Rolling; sometimes you need it before, sometimes after, sometimes both.

Supposing a man wants hard abs with muscle definition, but his posture is slumped, with head dropped forward and a concave chest. A workout program that only tightened his abs would make this pattern worse. Before he starts doing crunches, he needs to create length in the front of his torso, lifting his rib cage so his posture becomes more upright. He can do this by starting his workout with the Body Rolling abdominal routine.

If You Rarely Exercise

Perhaps you're always on the go, don't have any fitness regimen, and don't particularly want one. You feel fine, and that's enough for you. Body Rolling is a terrific way to maintain the level of fitness you need to keep you going. Because Body Rolling is so easy to incorporate into your life, it doesn't take much time. And even if you feel pretty good already, as Kathy discovered, Body Rolling can boost that feeling in surprising ways.

Marjorie was a real Type-A personality: stressful job, constantly active. She had a lot of energy, loved her lifestyle, and generally felt great, but she did feel tension accumulating every day in her neck and shoulders. She went for massages and took yoga classes, but the tension was always there. After her first Body Rolling session, however, she couldn't believe how relaxed her neck and shoulders were. "I feel like I rolled out my whole week!" she exclaimed. "It feels so good— better than a massage—and I can do it myself!"

And if you happen to be really out of shape—to the point where you have trouble doing things you want to do—but you just can't get motivated to exercise, even the simple Body Rolling routines that you can do in a chair watching TV or at your desk will improve your posture, boost your energy, strengthen your muscles, and increase your flexibility. Once you've reached this level of "better," you'll find that you want to try some new activities—maybe even going to the gym!

Beyond the Physical

A beautiful thing about Body Rolling is that, although it consists of a series of physical routines, its effects go way beyond your body to benefit your mind as well. That's because the physical improvements

Body Rolling produces translate into feeling better about yourself in general.

Like many women, Robin believed that in order to look thin she had to hold her stomach in all the time. She worried constantly about whether her stomach looked flat enough. After a while, keeping her abdominal muscles contracted became such a habit that she wasn't even aware she was doing it. But when you hold your stomach in, you can't breathe deeply, so Robin became a shallow breather with a tense, restricted rib cage and shoulders.

It wasn't until she did the Body Rolling abdominal routine that Robin finally took a deep breath for the first time in years. Lying over the ball made her breathe right into the area she was so used to holding in. As the ball pressed into her abdomen and she felt her muscles release, Robin realized how much that holding pattern had become ingrained in her—almost a part of her identity. When she finished the routine and stood up, she felt an amazing freedom in her pelvis, rib cage, and whole torso. And she actually felt high (and a bit lightheaded) from taking in so much more oxygen.

But what really astounded her was that she now had the look she'd wanted all along—taller, longer, and leaner. And she'd gotten it by doing the *opposite* of what she'd done all those years: elongating those contracted muscles instead of pulling them in. Robin told me she felt "liberated" by this tremendous improvement in her level of well-being, and her delight spilled over into everything she did. She felt more self-confident and more positive about life in general, and as a result found herself interacting more effectively with everyone she knew. Other people noticed a difference, too: she looked brighter, more alive and energetic. In fact, once you release a pattern of contraction that you've been holding all your life, every part of you functions better; even your skin color changes, since more oxygen is circulating through your body.

I see changes like these all the time in my clients. Once your neck and head are more relaxed, you can think more clearly. Once your neck and shoulders are light and free, the world no longer sits so heavily on them, and you lose that sense of pressure you might have carried around for years. Once your posture improves, your body moves more freely, so it's easier to do whatever you need to do. You feel better in your own skin, which makes you more relaxed and gives you self-assurance and, like Robin, an improved outlook on life.

EMOTIONAL RELEASE WITH BODY ROLLING

Sometimes, as you roll through tight areas of your body, you feel a tremendous sense of relief when your muscles release, and your whole being feels lighter afterward, as though a burden has been lifted. The chances are that in those areas you were holding old tension patterns that your body took on at some point. Such patterns are often rooted in some emotional issue and can get stuck in your body for years.

Emotional tension patterns are distinct from tension patterns that result from poor posture habits, and in fact they can compound other patterns. Emotional patterns vary: some people tighten their stomach, others start to itch, grow hot, or clench their jaw. Some sleep too much, others have insomnia. We tend to associate emotions with certain areas of the body: the chest or heart, the abdomen, throat, or lower back. But emotions can get lodged in some surprising places. One unexpected place that holds emotion is the armpit. Years of clenching their shoulders tightly to the side of their body have made the armpit an emotional storage area for many people.

Because the tensions we build up daily are often emotionally charged, releasing these tensions with regular Body Rolling keeps those emotions from getting stuck in the body and restricting us. For example, if the tension you hold in your body causes insomnia, by releasing that tension Body Rolling can help you sleep.

The good news is that you don't need to remember the exact experiences that might have caused an emotional tension pattern or to "process" them in order to release the tension. As you roll, the tension just melts out of your muscles and bones—and it stays out. Your body feels as though something that's been holding it back for years has suddenly let go.

Your Body Will Ask for More

Whenever I teach a workshop, I make an analogy between Body Rolling and psychotherapy. If during therapy you work on dysfunctional patterns that you have a habit of repeating, you develop an awareness that allows you to begin to break these patterns. You might still slip back into them occasionally, but since you now understand them, you can get out of them again. What happens with Body Rolling is similar. Once you've been doing it for a while, you'll find more and more that you can maintain the sense of greater ease and comfort you've developed. Your body has its own intelligence, and once it has the experience of feeling better, it wants to keep it. Even if you forget and fall back into your old pattern, your body will prod you back out of it. In fact, it's easier to change a body than a mind. That's why once you begin Body Rolling and experience the way it can affect every aspect of your being, you'll find that your body will always ask for more.

Body Rolling works for everyone, exercisers and non-exercisers alike. You can use it either to complement a fitness practice—yoga, martial arts, working with a trainer—or on its own. No matter who you are, Body Rolling will bring multiple transformations, as feeling better in your body brings a host of mental and emotional benefits. And you'll experience these truly amazing improvements starting with your very first session. I predict that whatever your own level of personal fitness is you'll wind up keeping Body Rolling in your life. Once you discover your own version of "better," you'll never let it go!

2

Understanding Your Body Architecture

Most of us, when we look in the mirror, see some part of our bodies that we wish looked different. Maybe we'd like a flatter stomach, a broader chest with muscle definition, or longer, leaner, sleeker thighs. So we put tremendous effort into trying to lose inches in this area or improve its shape. Then we're often frustrated to find we're not getting the changes we hoped for. But, in fact, you can change your shape more than you think—and it's *easy*. Frequently, it's simply a question of correcting your alignment—the way your bones, joints, and muscles fit together.

Gloria was an active gym-goer whose workouts resulted in big increases in her cardiovascular capacity and muscle tone. But nothing she tried could lift her sagging buttocks or reduce her wide hips and heavy thighs. Then her gym introduced Body Rolling as a new type of fitness class, and a friend insisted she try it. At her first class she did the routines for the buttocks and thigh muscles, then stood up. Her legs felt longer, and she could tell she was standing differently. But what really stunned Gloria was putting on her jeans after class and discovering that they were looser and hung better—the single buttocks routine had toned her derrière, so it was higher than before. On top of that, she actually looked thinner.

But the most important benefit Gloria received from Body Rolling was a direct experience of how specific muscles needed to change to enable her to get the sleek look she was after. For the first time, Gloria felt her gluteal (buttocks) muscles as a separate entity from her thighs. Instead of hanging down over her thighs, these muscles had suddenly perked up and started to function the way they were supposed to; that's why they were higher. And as Gloria rolled out her hips and thighs, her thigh muscles, which had been bunched up into her hips, began to elongate, so her thighs grew longer and thinner and her hips narrowed.

Few people realize that body alignment has any relation to how they look and feel, but the premise of Body Rolling is that if your body is properly aligned, your appearance will improve, any kind of physical activity will be easier, and your workouts will be more effective. That's why everybody who wants to be fit needs to understand the importance of what I call body architecture, by which I mean the alignment of bones, joints, and muscles, the structure that moves the body and takes you where you want to go. You need a solid structure that fully supports every part of your body. This means long, toned muscles; a spine that takes its maximum length; joints with adequate shock absorption and a full range of motion; and proper alignment.

To understand body architecture, you need to know how shock absorption is built into the human form. Every joint (the place where one bone meets another) contains cartilage, a spongy tissue that cushions the joint so that the bones slide past each other easily as you move. Years of simply walking with bones and muscles that aren't properly aligned will start to wear away the cartilage in your joints as the daily impact of your feet hitting the ground is transmitted upward to your ankles, knees, hips, and back. The uncushioned bones then rub against each other as you move, creating friction that wears them down. On the other hand, when your muscles are long and toned, there is adequate space in your joints, and your cartilage and bones are protected.

Imagine living in a building that's not architecturally sound. Many things can go wrong, from the foundation slipping to floors and walls shifting. Your body is your building, and all your parts need to be properly aligned, so that the whole structure can stand up over time. If your architecture is sound, your body will never let you down or hold you back from living to the fullest. We tend to accept physical limitations because they develop so slowly that we become used to them. But if you can't turn your head easily to look over your shoulder, or can't rotate your arm all the way behind you, that means your body architecture is holding you back.

On the same principle, whatever your form of workout is, if you don't have a sound architecture, you won't get the most out of your workout and might eventually injure yourself. And most of us do have some faulty architecture, whether it's the result of a hobby, our work, or our daily habits. Somebody who sits at his desk with rounded shoulders and head forward and then does an upper body routine at the gym in the evening could eventually hurt his shoulders or neck if he brings that work posture into his workout. A woman with one shoulder habitually hitched higher up than the other (usually from carrying a heavy bag) might hurt herself doing yoga postures that require shoulder stability. She's so used to this contraction that she doesn't realize that this shoulder stays lifted even when she's not carrying the bag. Then, when she tries to stretch both shoulders equally in yoga class, she's likely to injure a tendon or get a muscle spasm in the tight shoulder.

To me, the first step toward fitness is getting your structure well aligned so that it will last your entire lifetime. But people tend to focus on being "as strong as I can be" or burning calories. Our fitness culture is pervaded by a mentality of always needing to do more, which often leads people to push themselves too hard, especially with regard to cardiovascular exercise. I see more breakdown of body architecture from cardiovascular workouts than from exercise such as yoga, because people tend to do cardiovascular exercise mindlessly. They run or use the treadmill or stationary bicycle while reading or listening to music, paying no attention to their alignment during this intense activity. Instead, most are focused on keeping their heart in shape or burning calories so they can lose weight.

Most common knee, ankle, and hip injuries are caused by repetitive stress from cardiovascular exercise, because the repeated contraction of the muscles tightens and wears out the joints. Whether you're using cardiovascular exercise to warm up for your workout, or your cardiovascular routine is your whole workout, doing Body Rolling first to warm up and align your muscles will prevent this type of injury. What's more, if you use Body Rolling to free restrictions before any type of workout such as lifting weights, running, practicing yoga, or playing tennis, it's much easier to achieve correct form, as well as prevent injury.

For non-exercisers, whose faulty alignment comes from habitual poor posture (see "Repetitive Stress," later in this chapter), Body Rolling will reverse habits that could lead to discomfort in the future. Susan was a computer programmer who worked out at a gym and was generally in great shape. Being intelligent and well read, she knew that sitting for hours in front of a computer couldn't be good for her. She heard about Body Rolling and thought it sounded interesting, so she came to one of my classes.

We began by building length in the front of the body with the routines for the front of the pelvis and the chest (see chapters 5 and 9). When she finished and stood up, Susan was astonished to find that she felt "like a new person." She hadn't realized just how much her chest, head, and shoulders had been slumping forward toward the computer screen. The routines had released her tight chest muscles, letting her shoulders drop down and back and allowing her chest to open. Susan felt a new freedom in her body; she said she could breathe and even see better. "I'm truly shocked—I had absolutely no idea how radically different I could feel," she told me. "Being straight now makes me realize that I was totally unaware of how concave I was."

I see revelations like Susan's over and over. People get up from a session on the ball and exclaim, "I thought I was fine, but now I feel totally different! I'm seeing the world from a completely new place!" That's why a major message of this book is: even if you think you're perfectly okay now, you can always improve your body architecture somewhere—and doing so will have a wonderful effect on your entire being.

So how do you know whether your own architecture is solid? You start by learning to look at your own body alignment. Body Rolling teaches you to perceive what your body needs and gives you a tool to create the changes it's asking for—problem-finding and problem-solving together in one package. Like Susan, once your body is properly aligned, you'll breathe better, your organs will function better, and your body will move more easily. Most important, you'll be aware of how it feels to be straight, so when you start to slump, you can quickly correct your posture.

How Do We Lose Proper Alignment?

Nobody has perfect alignment. All of us have our own personal history: our activities as kids, the way we imitated our parents' posture. But two basic causes underlie all poor alignment patterns. The first is repetitive stress, which in my definition means any action you do repetitively over time—including many habitual motions of daily life.

The second is that most of us don't listen to the messages our bodies give us saying that something doesn't feel right.

REPETITIVE STRESS

People are increasingly conscious of repetitive stress syndrome as a hazard in the workplace or in sports. But repetitive stress goes beyond that. Every day we perform many actions unconsciously, and over time they become layered into the body and cause restrictions. If you habitually stand with your weight on one leg or chew on one side your whole life (some people do) or always cross the same leg over the other, you're setting up a pattern that your body will eventually get stuck in. Whether you're sitting in front of a computer, standing behind a counter all day, talking for hours with the phone always held to the same side of your head, or carrying your child constantly on the same arm, you're creating structural imbalances that gradually become ingrained in the body. These actions that you take for granted today are likely to contribute to a postural problem that could affect you ten or twenty years in the future.

Even the way you deal with ordinary stress is translated into the body as repetitive patterns. Some people contract their chest and constrict their breathing; others get stomach cramps, clench their jaw, or grind their teeth; still others develop neck pain. Often people develop a stress pattern like this during a difficult period in their life. Even after the difficulty passes, the pattern remains, then reemerges the next time they're under stress.

I believe that these tension patterns are as much a source of repetitive stress as computer keyboarding or playing tennis. Over time, they cause structural problems. People usually don't connect specific discomforts with this type of repetitive stress, so when I point out, "Do you know you clench your teeth?" they might respond, "Oh, yes, my dentist told me that"—but they've never realized that's why their neck and shoulders are so tight.

Start asking yourself how you use your body during your most mundane activities, so you can become aware of your own patterns and change them. For example:

- How do I use my body when I'm concentrating at my desk?

- Do I tend to lean forward in my chair? (If you do, make a point of leaning backward every now and then.)

- Do I stand with all my weight on one leg while washing dishes?

- Do I always carry groceries with the same arm?

Once we become aware of these patterns, it's often very simple to figure out how to change them. The moment I say to a client, "What's your pattern at work that makes you twist to the right all the time?" he realizes that's where the filing cabinet is, and it's been that way for years. Many structural problems arise out of simple daily movements like this. What's great is that you don't have to repeat these physical patterns—just as with psychological patterns, once you understand them you can break them and readjust the way you move your body. If you don't, you risk developing more serious structural problems, and possibly pain, down the line.

So take the time to examine those areas of your life where you perform the many unconscious movements that can get stuck in your body architecture. With Body Rolling, you can literally roll them out of your body—and your life!

IGNORING YOUR BODY'S MESSAGES

While Body Rolling can help you relieve structural problems, you have to start by paying attention to their warning signals. The first sign that something is wrong is restricted movement. Its message is: Stop and assess how you use whatever part of the body is holding you back. People commonly try to tough it out. They say, "I'm so busy, I

don't have time for this. Anyway, it's not that bad—I can deal with it."
They figure they'll just do nothing and wait a while to see if it gets
better.

But this approach is seriously wrong. Don't wait until the restriction leads to pain! Do something the moment you feel it. If you can't
raise your arm above your head, and you do nothing about it, your
shoulder is not going to loosen up—it's going to grow tighter. Eventually it will start restricting the areas around it—your neck and elbow. But when you find yourself with a stiff neck or an elbow that
gives you a twinge every time you move it, you aren't likely to connect that with your earlier shoulder problem. That's because, like
most of us, you were never taught that such relationships exist, that
one unstable piece of your body architecture can destabilize other
parts of your structure over time.

Another client of mine, Betsy, kept her computer on the right side
of her desk, since most of the time she needed to spread papers out in
front of her. When she did use the computer, her whole torso twisted
to the right. Eventually she noticed that when she stood up after a
day's work, her body remained in a rightward twist. Turning to face
straight forward required a conscious effort and no longer felt natural.

Fortunately, once Betsy realized what was happening, she began
to use Body Rolling to correct her alignment—and got a movable
arm to hold her computer monitor so she could position it straight in
front of her when she needed it, then push it away. If she hadn't fixed
her alignment pattern, her body would have stiffened into it. Eventually she'd have difficulty turning to the left. In the end, her body
would lose its memory of what facing forward while standing felt like.
She'd notice that she couldn't straighten herself out and wonder why.

It's essential, therefore, to pay attention to your body's messages,
as Betsy did when she came to me after noticing how she twisted to
the right. Once the message registers, you can begin to look for habitual actions you're not fully aware of that may be related. Just as
Betsy realized, "Gee, maybe it's the way I sit when I use the computer,"

you can notice how you might be sitting, consider how that might affect your body, then figure out a better sitting posture. In my experience, people often don't ask themselves those questions until something starts to hurt.

Don't wait until something unpleasant hits you over the head. By learning the few simple concepts presented in this book, you'll be able to understand what your body needs and prevent much discomfort, and even pain, that could be caused by your patterns of work, exercise, and daily habits. Body Rolling empowers you to care for your own structure. The easy routines in the following chapters are not just essential before embarking on any type of physical activity—they'll keep you youthful and pain-free in every sphere of life.

Learning the Language of the Body

When you feel a twinge during the day and think, "Gee, my neck's a little tight," or "My knees hurt a bit when I bent down," or "My back hurt when I did that stretch in yoga class," remember that this twinge is your body speaking to you, saying, "Something in that position or movement just then was not right for me!" Most of us are tempted to ignore the twinge and go on with whatever we're doing. So the next twinge will be stronger—your body trying a bit harder to communicate. How strong will the message have to get before you pay attention?

Joe, a serious cyclist, began to feel a tightness in the outside of his left knee. It usually came on after riding and lasted through the next day. The moment he got on his bike and started riding again it felt better, so he figured he was doing the right thing to loosen it up. This went on for several months, until one day, cycling up a steep hill that required strong exertion, he heard something pop in that knee. He iced it, but it still felt a bit sore. When he woke the next day, his knee was quite inflamed and painful, and he couldn't walk on it. He went to a doctor, who recommended knee surgery.

Joe's body had been giving him messages all along that something he was doing was making his knee unhappy, but like most people, he imagined he was "working through it" and that with time, the problem would work itself out. But in fact, "working itself out" is a concept that does not apply to the body. You can't just leave a body problem alone—you must do something specific to take care of it, even if that something is simply to stop doing whatever is hurting you or figure out a better way to do it. If you keep ignoring your body's messages, it repeats them louder, which is to say with more pain and discomfort. Unheeded, the pain eventually becomes chronic. Most injuries, like Joe's, occur simply because people didn't listen to the body's initial warning signs. These physical sensations are the language of the body, and understanding that language is the key to feeling good as well as preventing serious problems.

Julie was a computer programmer who spent hours staring at the screen each week. She was always irritable and exhausted, complaining of floaters and black spots before her eyes, as well as constant shoulder and neck pain with a burning sensation down into her hands. Julie knew very well that her body was screaming at her and that the stress at her job was the reason for its distress, but she didn't feel she could change anything at the office. Her job involved a lot of responsibility and tremendous pressure, but she loved it just the same. What she could do, however, was take a look at how her work was affecting her body and figure out how to improve her posture.

First, Julie made sure she wasn't leaning forward into the computer. Instead, she focused on keeping her head, neck, shoulders, and back in a straight line, resting against her chair. She also remembered to keep track of the level of tension in her hands and use less pressure on the keys. And she used Body Rolling to release the poor alignment patterns that her working habits had created in her shoulders, chest, and back. Listening to her body's messages, then responding appropriately, prevented Julie from developing a repetitive stress injury that might have kept her from working at all.

THE BODY-MIND DIALOGUE

As Kathy discovered in chapter 1, a wonderful benefit of Body Rolling is the way it sharpens your awareness of how the different parts of your body feel. The moment Kathy realized that her right side was tighter than the left, her mind started working to figure out how she used the right side differently. This is an example of what I call the body-mind dialogue: listening to the language of the body, which consists of physical sensations; responding to these messages by paying attention to them; then using your mind to understand what's happening in your body.

Supposing your habitual posture is a slouch. If you do the Body Rolling routine for the front of the body, rolling up your chest while lying on the ball, you immediately feel a new sensation: your rib cage moves upward, away from your abdomen, and as you inhale, you feel your chest expanding against the ball. When you finish and stand up, you sense your body moving into a new, more upright posture. Now your body knows what standing up straight feels like, and you know what changes are necessary to make that happen.

Here's a more sophisticated example. In yoga class, you've been practicing Seated Angle Pose (a variation of the forward bend in which your legs are stretched wide to each side as you try to lower your torso to the floor between them). No matter how you try, you've never gotten very far. But while doing Body Rolling on your inner thighs, you suddenly have the insight that the muscles there are the ones that need to stretch in order to do that yoga pose. So you finish rolling out those muscles and try the pose. Amazingly, you get four or five inches closer to the floor than ever before—plus, when you stand up, your groin muscles feel lubricated, and you experience a new ease in walking.

By teaching you how to think about your own structure, Body Rolling gives you a whole new way of being in your body. Often, when people experience restriction or pain in their bodies, they immediately assume they have to go to a health-care practitioner to learn what's wrong with them. But when I ask people who come to me with specific restrictions they want to release, "What do you think is really going on?" they can generally tell me in very simple language exactly what it is. With a little prompting, if I ask how they sit when they work or what their sport or hobby is, they can also figure out the cause. Most of the time, if you just listen to your own perceptions, you'll find that you know what the problem is.

Suppose that when you're sitting in your chair at work, your lower back always hurts on the left side. So, following my basic back routine, you roll up the two sides of your spine. As you roll, you notice that the sides of your back feel quite different. The left side feels fairly loose and easy, but the right side is tight and contracted; there's discomfort all the way up. Your mind wonders: "I always hurt on the left, so why is the right side so tight?"

When you finish the routine and stand up, you discover that the left side doesn't hurt anymore. The mind wants to understand this, so it goes to work and figures out that the imbalance between the two sides—with the right so much tighter—could be what caused the pain on the left. The next question is: "If I keep the right side more stretched out, will the pain on the left go away?" The answer—which you can discover for yourself by using the ball to release contraction on the right side—is yes. With this new ability to communicate with your body, you'll find a whole universe of wonderful improvements you can achieve on your own.

Joe, the cyclist, waited until his injury healed, then used the ball to roll from his pelvis to his knees on the front, back, and sides of both thighs. He noticed that the sensation from the ball was far more intense on the outside of his left thigh—the side with the injured knee—than on the inside of the same thigh. So he realized that those outside muscles were much tighter than the inside ones. This discovery led him to wonder whether this tightness was affecting his knee. He asked himself, "What am I doing as I ride to make those muscles so tight?"

The next time he rode, he watched where his knees were in relation to his hips and feet, and saw that they were turned out to the side, but the left knee was more turned out than the right. Then the light flashed. Joe realized that he'd been riding this way throughout his cycling career, developing an alignment pattern that caused his injury. So he began making a conscious effort as he cycled to keep his knees parallel to each other. Meanwhile he continued to use the ball to keep all his thigh muscles equally elongated, and the inner and outer thigh muscles balanced, so he could completely heal his injury and prevent another one.

While preventing injury is certainly important, the knowledge you get from Body Rolling goes beyond that. Your increased awareness makes you generally smarter about how you use your body. Once you begin standing taller, you're aware that this posture feels better, so your body begins to assume it more often. You might be reading on the bus, catch yourself in your old position of hunching forward, and immediately sit up straight, because that now feels easier and better. In the same way, people who used to put all their weight on one foot begin distributing their weight on both feet, because that now feels better. If you lift weights, once Body Rolling has helped you develop the sensation of what square shoulders and a broad chest feel like, you'll bring that feeling into your weight lifting, so you'll no longer be doing your workout with rounded shoulders. Once you've learned the language of the body, it takes very little time and effort to maintain that communication and keep your body happy.

Analyzing Your Body Architecture

When we're children, we learn certain ways to care for our bodies, to brush our teeth and comb our hair in the morning, for example. But no one teaches us to look at where our shoulders are today, how our neck is, and so on. Yet this kind of well-developed body awareness is something everyone can have—something you yourself can and should develop, starting today, with Body Rolling. You look in the mirror every day, so why not take that opportunity to check out your structure? You can see a lot more than you might imagine.

My First Self-Analysis

I first looked in the mirror myself because I had a structural problem that experts couldn't solve. When my daughter was born, the impact of the delivery tore the inner thigh muscles of my left leg. These muscles help hold the leg in the hip joint, so without them, my thighbone kept getting dislocated from its socket. I couldn't walk, and I was in a lot of pain. I went to a whole range of body therapists, but nothing worked. Then, on my way home after three months of expensive visits to a chiropractor who would adjust the thighbone back into place, I stepped off a curb and it dislocated again. I came home disgusted and—for the first time—looked in the mirror.

Observing my own architecture, I was shocked to see how different my left and right legs looked. In contrast to the right leg, the left one just hung there. The left inner thigh muscles were obviously not supporting the leg at all. My knee and ankle were collapsed. Without knowing anything about how the left leg was supposed to look, just by comparing it to the right leg, I could see how unstable it was.

For the first time in my life, my mind started working to try to figure out what was happening in my body. I said to myself, "Let *me* find the solution. If those inner thigh muscles are so weak, they must not be working. So what can I do to get them to work?"

I was a yoga teacher, so I applied my yoga knowledge to the problem. Examining the leg, I realized that the outside thigh muscles had become extremely tight, since they were working so hard to compensate for the weakness of the inner thigh. So I set to work to release that tightness. I did yoga postures that stretched the outside thigh muscles. Releasing the tightness on the outside, I figured, would allow the inner muscles to regain their function. Once that was accomplished, I did stretches that toned the inner muscles until they became strong enough to hold my thighbone in the hip socket.

This story shows just how valuable the mirror can be. And you don't have to master a complicated form of analysis or learn anatomy. Most people observing their structure in the mirror will see some difference between the two sides of their body, even when they don't have any body problem. This difference gives your mind a clue, so it can start thinking about what you do in your life that might create this difference—and about what you can do to make both sides equal. The information you get from the mirror is particularly useful when you're experiencing some discomfort that you want to relieve or when you'd like to improve the way a particular part of you looks. Then, once you use Body Rolling to work on the relevant areas, the mirror tells you that you've succeeded. Once you see how easy it is to create improvements, you'll be eager to see how many other changes are possible, and you'll keep on rolling.

What Is Optimal Posture?

Whether you have a body problem to figure out or you just want to keep yourself in good alignment, you need to start by knowing what optimal posture is.

Generally speaking, when your body is properly aligned your weight is distributed so that standing is effortless. Since you're not leaning either forward or backward, no muscles have to contract anywhere in your body to hold you up, as they do when your body isn't balanced. You stand fully upright, and no part of your body feels restricted.

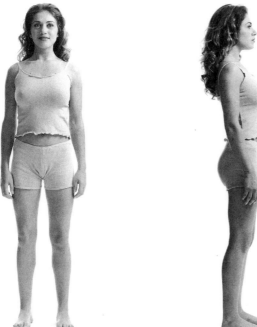
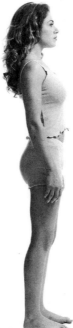

Optimal posture, front view   **Optimal posture, side view**

Here are some specific points to be aware of:

- Your feet face straight forward; they're not turned in or out.

- Your ankles are straight, not collapsed inward or outward.

- Your pelvis is centered, not tilted forward or backward.

- Your torso and spine are erect, lifting upward, not collapsing down. Your chest is lifted; it doesn't drop into the abdomen.

- Your shoulders, neck, and head are in the same line. The shoulders aren't rotated forward, and the head doesn't jut out in front of the shoulders.

Now, keeping these points in mind, stand facing a full-length mirror and try a simple exercise.

Am I Standing as Tall as I Can?

The chances are that as soon as you ask yourself this question, you'll make yourself stand up straighter. So notice which parts of you get lifted or repositioned when you do this. Commonly people tighten their knees, lift their shoulders and rib cage, and move their head back. This shows you right away all the parts you need to adjust in order to stand up straight and tells you that all these areas are restricting you day-to-day. You might already have some developing discomfort in them. But even if they feel perfectly fine, it's still a good idea to start correcting them right away.

With this exercise you've already accomplished the first step in discovering how your body architecture can improve. In chapters 4 through 9, you'll learn how to look at the separate parts of your body to see where you may have other misalignments that you can correct with specific Body Rolling routines. And even if you aren't always completely sure about what you see in the mirror, don't worry—Body Rolling will improve your alignment *automatically.*

Remember that nobody can stay perfectly conscious of their body all the time. We tend to get involved in whatever we're doing and forget about our posture. But you can develop the habit of checking in with your body periodically. If you find yourself falling into an old pattern, just get on the ball and roll it right out of your muscles. The next chapter will give you all the information you need to get rolling right away.

3

Getting on the Ball

Now you're ready to get rolling! You won't believe how a practice that can be so transformative is also so easy. No matter who you are, you can integrate Body Rolling into your lifestyle. Since you can practice it almost anywhere, it will enhance everything you do. Start your morning with it, then keep rolling all day long. The guidelines that follow in this chapter will ensure that you get the most out of Body Rolling.

Choosing the Right Ball

Choosing a ball that's right for your body is extremely important for achieving the results you want. Using the right ball will also prevent you from getting hurt.

Based on feedback from my clients, I spent several years designing a series of special balls that work best for Body Rolling. These re-inflatable balls have the right density, resistance, and weight-bearing capacity for different types of bodies. The more you let yourself sink into one of these balls, the more deeply it will press into your body. Because my balls enable you to clearly feel differences between muscles, they make it much easier to work on specific muscles that are tight. These balls also exert the right degree of pressure to change the quality of bone. You can deflate and reinflate them when traveling, and they'll last for years. (See Resources, page 213, for mail-order information.) What's more, all my balls can hold up to 350 pounds, making Body Rolling available to everyone.

When I first created Body Rolling, I used the inexpensive vinyl children's balls found in drugstores. Most people can try Body Rolling using one of these balls, but—though you'll certainly get some benefits—vinyl balls lack adequate density and resistance and cannot be reinflated. Inflatable utility balls, available at toy stores or sporting goods stores, are denser and more durable, and you can adjust their hardness. But you won't get the very best results and deepest muscle releases with either of these types of balls. Moreover, anyone weighing over 180 pounds cannot use them because the balls will bend out of shape and not provide any benefit at all.

The Yamuna® Body Rolling Balls

Yellow ball. I recommend that everyone begin Body Rolling with my yellow ball, which is made of soft plastic that's comfortable for your body to sink into. Anyone can do all the Body Rolling routines safely with this ball, and most people will also find it the best one for abdominal work.

Red ball. This is a harder ball, which most people can work up to using for all the routines (except possibly for abdominal routines). It lets you sink more deeply into muscles, for more intense work. However, people over sixty; those with fibromyalgia, osteoarthritis, osteoporosis, or other bone abnormalities; and anyone who has recently had surgery or is in rehab after an injury should not use this ball. Also, people who retain a great deal of fluid in their legs are likely to find it too painful and should stick with the yellow ball for leg routines.

Green ball. This ball has the same consistency as the yellow ball but is smaller, so it can get into areas like the neck and armpits or between the breasts. Shorter people can use it instead of the yellow ball on the abdomen, although since it's smaller it goes in deeper, so the sensation is generally more intense. This ball is also intended for use in the workplace, against the wall or the back of your chair, and for traveling. You can use it on an airplane, in a car, or on a train without bothering the person next to you. I also recommend it for children and for general use by adults under five feet.

Yamuna® Ball Care

To pump up your ball, first wet the pump needle, then insert it straight into the valve. If the needle doesn't go in easily, you're probably pushing it against the side of the valve. Don't push hard—you may puncture the valve and ruin the ball. Instead, change the angle of the needle. Inflate the ball to the point where you can press into it with your fingers and easily produce a slight indentation. Don't inflate it so much that you can't do this. Overinflation will stretch the plastic and change its resistance.

Keep your ball away from radiators and out of direct sunlight, since heat and sunlight will soften the plastic; once the ball softens it won't stay hard as long and will increase in size when reinflated. I can't tell you the exact size each ball should be, for the size changes depending on the atmosphere. Fully inflated balls will be larger in a hot, humid climate than in a cold climate, not because they're damaged but because heat and humidity affect the elasticity of the plastic. What's important is getting the right degree of hardness.

BALLS FOR THE FEET

You can also do Body Rolling on your feet, but for the foot routines you need a different ball, called a sponge ball. It should be about two and a half inches in diameter and made of solid rubber that's firm, not soft. Among the solid balls that are available, the best I have found is the Pinky, sold at drugstores and chain stores such as Kmart and Wal-Mart. You will need two balls so you can work both feet at the same time.

- *Don't use a golf ball or Superball on your feet.* **These balls are far too hard** *and will injure you.*

- ***Don't use a tennis ball or any other hollow ball.* Instead of giving like solid rubber, a hollow ball will indent when you put all your weight into it.**

I've also developed "Foot Savers," plastic half-spheres with flat bottoms that are easier to balance on than balls. Foot Savers allow you to work all the points of the foot in much greater detail. (For mail-order information, see Resources, page 213.)

What to Wear

For Body Rolling you need comfortable clothing without zippers, snaps, or belts. Close-fitting exercise clothes work best. The ball tends to get caught in loose clothing, and bulky garments such as sweatshirts make it difficult to feel exactly where the ball is. Men usually prefer wearing some kind of top, since the ball can pull chest or back hair. Also, if it's hot and you perspire, the ball can stick to your skin or slip. Avoid slick fabrics, which will slide right off the ball.

Where to Practice

It's most comfortable to do Body Rolling with some kind of padding on the floor, such as an exercise mat or carpet. Towels or blankets don't work because they slip around and bunch up. A yoga sticky mat helps prevent the ball from slipping out from under you and gives your feet extra traction for some of the routines.

You can also practice against a wall, in your office chair, watching TV, or anyplace that's convenient. I travel a lot, and I've been known to do Body Rolling on the floor in airports!

How Long Does It Take?

People always say they don't have time—it's the biggest complaint I hear. But in fact, you always have time. You always have five minutes to work on yourself—especially if that five minutes can make a big difference. Here are some of the things you can do in five minutes:

- If your knees or hamstrings feel tight, you can roll out the back of your thighs (pages 105–109).

- If you have neck tension, you can roll up your spine and the back of your neck (pages 60–68), or do the back of the neck routine by itself (pages 146–50).

- If you're sitting at your office desk and notice that you're hunched forward, you can do the chest routine against the wall (pages 178–80).

People tend to slot "working on my body" into the time they spend at the gym or in an exercise class, but you can do Body Rolling at many other times. For most routines I offer a complete, detailed version—which gives you the most benefits and takes the longest to do—plus one or more modifications for doing the routine in other settings and other positions and in less time. You won't get the same results as you would from the full routines, but the variations will definitely provide quick relief.

You'll soon figure out lots of places in your life where you can fit in Body Rolling. Often you find yourself sitting somewhere for a period of time and instead of doing nothing you can work on yourself. I find that many people use the ball more at work than at home. They keep it against their chair back all day to counter their tendency to hunch forward or move it under their legs as they work (see the routines on pages 75–76 and 118–21). My clients tell me that doing Body Rolling in the office actually improves the quality of their work. It enhances their sitting position and leaves them less tired at the end of the day, since preventing your muscles from getting tight and restricted gives you more energy. Plus, they love the fact that they're getting their workout while they work.

Always remember that—even with a five-minute routine—it's important to be fully present as you do it. Take the time to breathe properly at each point (see the section on breathing, later in the chapter) and wait until you feel your body really sinking into the ball before you move to the next point. If you race through a routine, you won't get the full benefit.

Basic Rules of Body Rolling

The following rules are important for two reasons. First, they're essential safety precautions. Second, by following them you'll ensure that the routines produce the effects you're looking for.

- **If you've ever had an accident, been injured, or had surgery, or if you suffer from chronic pain or experience a sudden severe pain anywhere in your body, consult a health-care professional before beginning Body Rolling.**

- **Always do the routines in the specified order.** One reason Body Rolling is so effective is that it's based on the body's logic and order: starting where the muscle begins, rolling toward where it ends. Rolling back and forth simply doesn't have the same effect.

- **Always do a routine on *both* sides of the body, even if only one side hurts.** When you have discomfort on one side of your body, your natural tendency is to focus there. But since what's causing the problem is how the two sides work together, you need to work both of them. And if you roll out just one side, you leave the other side confused. Its reaction is to contract, introducing a new negative posture pattern. Instead, you want to keep the two sides balanced and symmetrical. This rule applies to the legs and arms as well as the torso.

- **Remember that sinking into the ball with all your weight doesn't mean *pushing* into the ball.** Let your body *sink*—don't try to push or pull it down. This is not a "no pain, no gain" exercise—it's about staying fit by *letting go.*

- *At all times* **avoid rolling near the lowest rib on each side (called the "floating rib") and the rib right above it.** These ribs are very easily broken, so avoid exerting any pressure anywhere near them.

- **Don't roll into an area that is swollen or inflamed.** You can roll above and below that area, but don't put any direct pressure on the swelling or inflammation.

- **Don't roll up the front of the abdomen to the ribs.** Again, it's easy to break a rib this way.

- **Never use *any* ball on the bottom tip of your breastbone; it is fragile and can easily break.** Make sure you place the ball at least an inch and a half from the very bottom of the breastbone.

Getting Comfortable on the Ball

For the regular Body Rolling routines, you'll be on the floor, sitting or lying on the ball. Most people need to begin by getting comfortable in this position, so I start my classes by showing people how to sit on the ball—and how to fall off. With this simple balancing exercise, you're already improving your balance and core strength.

Once you can sit on the ball comfortably, you'll easily figure out how to move around on it according to the directions in the routines. The following little exercise shows you how the mind is drawn to focus on the point of the body where the ball is. It is therefore the beginning of the body-mind dialogue.

Introduction to the Ball

1. Place the ball under your right sitbone, sinking all your weight into it. Use your hands or fingertips on the floor alongside your hips or a little behind you to help support you and for balance.

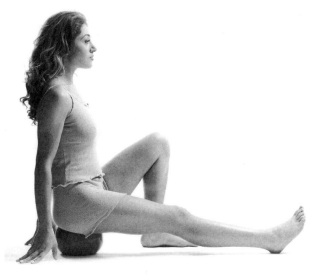

Step 1

Tip for step 1

*   *To find your sitbone, sit on your hands. You'll feel a bone about an inch and a half wide under each buttock. This is the sitbone, the lowest part of your pelvis. It is* not *your tailbone.*

2. Extend your right leg straight out in front of you, keeping the left leg bent. The left foot is flat on the floor, helping you balance and move on the ball. Use your hands or fingertips on the floor to help support you and for balance.

3. Gently move your body forward and backward so the ball rolls behind, then in front of, the sitbone. Use your fingertips and left leg to shift yourself two inches forward and two inches backward in a smooth, easy movement.

4. Using your fingertips and left leg, shift your body weight from side to side on the ball, building up momentum so the ball rolls off one end of the right sitbone, then back across it to the other end, and so on. These are micromovements; you're only rolling an inch or two in each direction.

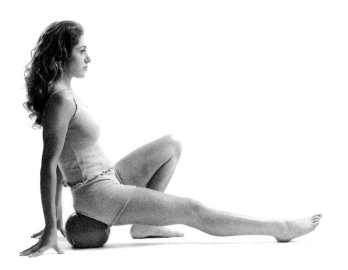

Step 3, rolling forward

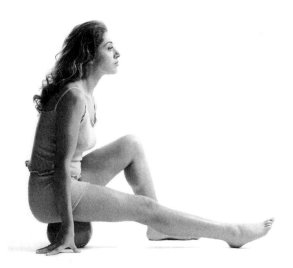

Step 3, rolling backward

5. Now shift your weight slightly more to the left and let the ball roll out from under you toward the right as you slide off it to the left. This shows you that falling off the ball is safe. You won't get hurt because you're not going very far.

6. Repeat on the left side, placing the ball under the left sitbone.

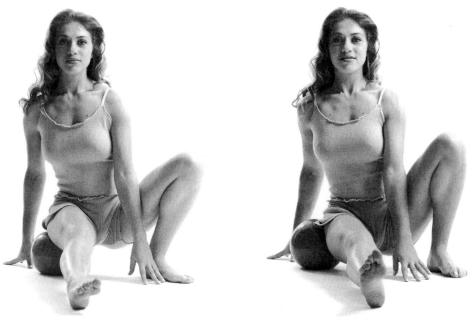

Step 4   Step 5

Where Do I Start?

It's natural to want to begin Body Rolling at a particular part of your body that's achy or stiff—and you can, if you like, go straight to the chapter that covers this area. But I suggest instead that you begin by getting your body used to the way Body Rolling feels, and the best way to do that is by practicing the basic back routine that starts on page 60. This is the routine that's most beneficial for your whole body. Starting with it gives you a chance to really feel comfortable on the ball; it builds balance and core strength; and releasing your back will make work on every other part of your body more effective.

If you don't feel particularly stiff anywhere, and what you want is general toning and flexibility, you should still begin with the back routine. Then, after you analyze your body architecture, if you discover a particular misalignment or see an area you'd like to create more space in, go to the chapter that covers that area. Or you can simply work your way through the routines for the entire body, one step at a time. Doing so provides a wonderful total-body workout.

If you have time, you'll always get the most benefit by starting or ending your session with the back routine. (Of course, it's great to both start *and* end with the back routine, but most people don't have *that* much time.) At the beginning of the session, releasing the back enables the rest of the body to release more easily. At the end, the back routine increases the length created by the other routines and helps hold the releases and realignment these other routines have achieved. For example, if you do the front and side routines, finishing with the back routine will hold and possibly even increase the length you've created in your torso.

The Flow of the Session Is the Flow of Your Breath

A big missing piece in most people's body education is that we don't learn about all the things our breath can do for our bodies. Body Rolling shows you how to direct your breathing to different areas and feel it go there. You'll begin to understand why deeper breathing is essential to achieve relaxation and you'll discover how you can use the breath to profoundly increase your well-being.

Yoga, martial arts, and other physical practices put great emphasis on proper breathing techniques. But with Body Rolling, you don't have to learn a technique to get the benefits of deep breathing. All you have to do is focus your breath wherever the ball is, as your torso expands against the ball as you inhale, then sinks into it as you exhale.

The general rule for pacing a Body Rolling session is to integrate your breathing with the movement of the ball. With the ball at a specific point, you inhale, feeling your body push out against it. Then you exhale, feeling the weight of your body sink into the ball. At the *end* of the exhale, you move the ball to the next point, then inhale again.

Generally, you take one full, deep breath at each point, then move to the next one. But at points where you particularly want to release tension, you may want to stay longer, using each inhale to expand further against the ball and each exhale to sink deeper into it. Many people store tension deep inside their bodies. Consciously engaging your lungs in the effort to push out against the ball and then letting go as you sink into it will release that deep tension. You'll feel your muscles soften as you use your breath this way. This effort tones the diaphragm and the muscles of the rib cage, giving the lungs more room to expand.

> *Remember: You're not in a rush.* At each point, breathe and *wait,* concentrating on a deep inhale and then a long, slow exhale as you let your tissue sink deeper into the ball. Staying for a full breath at each point gives your mind time to take in what is happening there.

If you follow these instructions, you'll find yourself naturally breathing more fully throughout your whole torso, even if you're normally a chest breather or an abdominal breather. In this way you increase your breathing capacity, your ribs become more flexible as your rib cage expands further, and your entire torso relaxes. People in my classes who do this breathing for the first time stand up and discover that their bodies are more open and they're breathing into parts of their torso that they didn't even realize their breath could reach.

Pacing with the breath is easy when you're working on the torso, since you can feel your inhalation push your body against the ball. Working on the legs, though, you don't feel the breath in the same way, but you can still use it to pace yourself. Focus on taking a full breath at each point; this will help you stay at that point long enough for your muscles to sink into the ball.

What Will It Feel Like?

The basic sensation in Body Rolling is one of pressure exerted by your body weight at the point where it sinks into the ball. This pressure then dissipates as the muscles and tendons there release and let go. As this release occurs, you feel yourself sink farther into the ball, and your body stretches more around it. At particularly tight areas in your body, you might find that this release doesn't happen at first. But if you stay at those points and continue to breathe, you'll start to feel the muscles soften and relax with each breath, and you'll begin to sink deeper into the ball. Then, when you stand up, you can see the physical change that this release has created, and you'll feel that part of your body moving more freely.

After you've been doing Body Rolling for a while, releases happen more easily. Doing the back routine, for example, you'll feel the back muscles letting go in a wave from the lower back up to the top as you roll. When the ball reaches your neck, you feel a continuing release as the jaw relaxes, the eyes relax, and the shoulders drop. You feel that if you continue to lie there, your body will keep sinking and sinking, as though it could go right through the floor and the sinking might never stop.

WHAT IF IT HURTS?

At some points, the pressure of your body weight on the ball can be painful as you press on tight, constricted muscles. This pain is an indication of how tense and tight that area is. What you should try to do, as much as you can, is remain at that point for another two or three breaths (using your arms and knees if necessary to support your weight, so the pressure on the ball stays at a level you can tolerate).

The pain will decrease, and the amount of that decrease is the measure of how much tension you have released.

If, however, you feel a sudden, *sharp* pain as you roll into an area (often the rib cage), instead of staying at this spot, immediately move the ball to the next point. Chances are that once you create length in this area as a whole, the next time you roll over that particular point you won't feel that sharp pain and will be able to remain there and breathe.

In the next few chapters, we'll take a closer look at each part of the body. You'll learn the basic routines and achieve a certain degree of release in each area. Once your body is used to Body Rolling, your muscles will let go faster. For example, for the first couple of weeks it may take you a half hour each day to get your back nice and open by doing the back routine. From this point on, however, you'll likely find that you only need five minutes a day to keep your back relaxed. You can then use the extra time to focus on other areas that you really want to work on, and go for your optimum release there.

Unlike fitness practices that require willpower and discipline, Body Rolling is self-motivating. All the routines are designed to give you noticeable results from the very first session. And they'll continue to work—as long as you do them the way I've described, using your breath to the fullest and giving yourself time to wait for the muscles to release, all the way to that deep, deep sink.

4

Your Basic Routine: Up the Back

The Body Rolling back routine is a wonderful way to energize yourself when you get out of bed in the morning. It will wake up your spine and roll out any little kinks or stiffness that remain after your night's sleep. You'll be in better shape for any activity—working, exercising at the gym, or getting your kids off to school. Body Rolling makes it easy to add back maintenance to your daily routines—and we all need to be good to our backs.

The back is the part of the body that most affects every other part. That's why it's essential to keep your spine healthy, and why the most important Body Rolling routine is the basic back routine. The back's powerful influence stems from the spine, which consists of a column of bones called vertebrae stacked on top of each other, running from the bottom of your tailbone up to your skull. Your spinal cord passes through a hole in the center of each vertebra. The roots of all your nerves emerge from the spinal cord and pass out between the vertebrae to almost every part of the body. When the spine is in distress, therefore, the entire body will be affected. A healthy spine requires adequate space between the vertebrae so that there is no pressure on the spongy disks that sit between them and act as little shock absorbers allowing the spine ample freedom of movement.

Bad posture, stress, strain, injury, and just plain gravity can cause the space between the vertebrae to decrease, squashing the disks. Under this pressure the disks begin to degenerate, and eventually they protrude outside the spinal column and press on nerves, causing pain (this condition is known as a slipped disk or bulging disk). If the disks are compressed over a long enough period of time, all the cushioning between the vertebrae is lost. The vertebrae start to grind against each other as you move, and the bone begins to wear away. Not only is your movement restricted, but the stage is set for osteoporosis, arthritis, and other bone disorders. But if you understand the importance of stretching out your back muscles, you can prevent all this from happening. So I urge you to add back maintenance to your daily routines.

To maintain the space between the vertebrae, you need toned, elongated back muscles that support the spine so it can take its full length. Most people have heard of the big muscles on the surface of the back, the trapezius and latissimus dorsi, which fitness buffs work on in the gym. But you may not be familiar with the powerful chain of tiny muscles that start at the base of the spine and run up to the skull. Their job is simply to stabilize and move the spine and to hold it upright so the vertebrae have the maximum amount of space. The trapezius and the latissimus dorsi are attached to the spine, and if the small muscles are very tight, they will contract those big muscles in toward the spine, constricting the movement of the hips, torso, and shoulders.

If you're a person who tends to hold tension in your back, the chances are that after years of being contracted those small muscles are so gripped to your spine that they keep it fairly rigid, preventing real flexibility and freedom of movement and cutting off adequate circulation to the nerve roots—thus affecting all your organs. Once you've become fairly stiff, many ordinary, everyday activities can contribute to a lower back problem: lifting heavy objects, getting in and out of cars, carrying heavy packages, vacuuming, moving furniture, coughing, sneezing, bending over to make the bed, even making love—all these activities can throw people's lower back out.

The basic back routine will keep those little muscles flexible; increase the tone, range of motion, and flexibility of the big back muscles; increase circulation; and improve your alignment so your posture is more upright. I've also included a routine for elongating the abdominal muscles which will bring relief when your lower back has been speaking to you with twinges and twitches.

People who have a history of back problems are often fearful about working on their backs. For them, I've added modifications of the basic routine, so pick the one you feel most comfortable doing.

Optimal Back Alignment

Our spine is made to be flexible and to change position according to the type of action we're engaged in. This means that there's no single optimal alignment for the back. So a healthy back is simply one that's flexible, strong, and as long as possible, with space between the disks. Such a back is erect—it doesn't slouch or curve to one side. It lets you perform any movement with ease and freedom.

These days, nobody has a perfectly aligned spine. Look around you: even people in their twenties are slouching. If they do nothing to correct this posture, in twenty years they'll be slouching even more. But with Body Rolling, you can easily keep your back flexible, long, and strong for years to come.

Self-Exam

This exercise will wake you up to postural habits that may be affecting your back. Since it's hard to look at your back in a mirror, much of the self-exam below involves observing daily actions.

- First, stand naturally in front of a mirror and observe yourself. Are you standing as tall as you can? Are you slouching anywhere? If you're slouching, can you straighten up?

- If you work sitting at a desk, how do you sit? Do you round your shoulders forward, pull your head forward, let your belly drop? This posture puts strain on your upper back and neck. Does your body lean or twist to one side to reach your computer or talk on the phone? Maintaining this pattern will eventually curve your spine permanently in that direction.

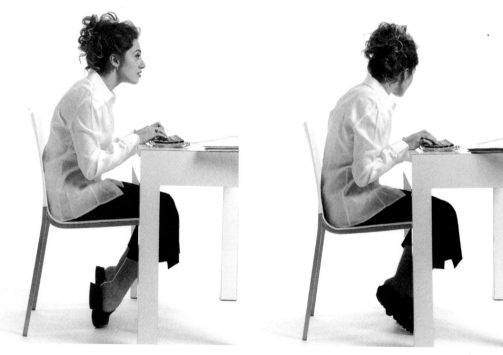

Shoulders rounded forward   **Body twisted to the side**

- If you stand on your feet all day for your job, do you let your torso slouch? Slouching creates a downward pressure that weakens your lower back.

- Notice how you walk. Are you heavy on your feet, elephant-like? Such a gait puts enormous pressure on your lower back, since the disks there are absorbing the force exerted upward by the pounding feet.

- Are your abdominal muscles toned or weak? Do you use them to help take the load off your back during lifting or exercise?

If you answer yes to any of the questions in the first four bullet points and you feel tightness, restriction, or discomfort in your spine, you've already begun to see how your daily activities may be contributing to back tension. The good news is that the following back routines will strengthen your back muscles and break your slouching pattern—whatever may be causing it.

The Basic Back Routine

If you're looking for a single general routine to do daily to keep your spine healthy, this is the one I recommend—especially since it also benefits your whole body. The basic back routine is done on the floor and gives the most powerful results. I've also included two variations to use in your office or whenever you can't get down on the floor: one uses the wall; the other is done in a chair and is great anytime you find yourself sitting for long periods of time.

Because tight hamstrings (the muscles along the backs of the thighs) can prevent you from achieving the greatest length in your spine, this basic routine starts with a gentle release of these muscles before you actually begin rolling up the back.

1. Place the ball under the right sitbone (for instructions on finding your sitbone, see page 49), with the right leg extended

straight out. Use your hands or fingertips on the floor to help support you and for balance. Bend the left knee up, keeping the left foot flat on the floor to help you to balance on the ball and to move. Roll the ball forward and backward, then side to side on the sitbone. Roll clockwise, then counterclockwise. Your right leg will bend a bit as you move the ball around the sitbone.

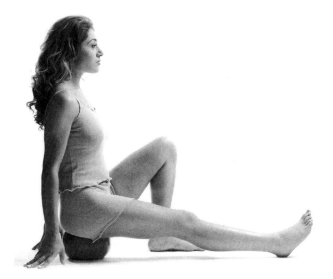

Step 1

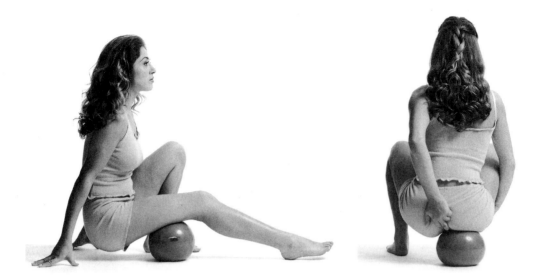

Step 2

Step 3

2. Using your fingertips and left foot, pull your body behind you and roll the ball a couple of inches down the back of your leg. Take a full breath in and let the ball sink into the back of your leg as you exhale, elongating the hamstrings. Roll the ball a couple of inches down the leg two or three more times, breathing and sinking each time. Stop when you're about two-thirds of the way to the knee. Then roll the ball back up to the sit-bone in one smooth movement.

Tip for step 2

- *Your fingertips move either in front of you or behind you to help you move the ball down your leg. The tighter your hamstrings are, the farther behind your torso your fingertips will be. If your hamstrings are more flexible, your fingertips might be beside your hips or even in front of them.*

3. Now you're ready to begin rolling up the back. With the fingers of your left hand, feel for the tailbone—the last bony piece

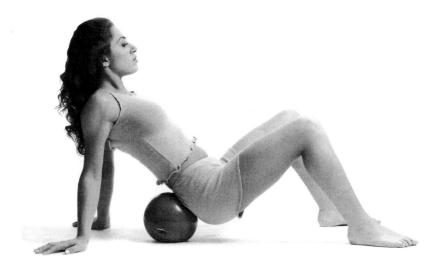

Step 5

of the spine that you can feel. Roll the ball from the right sit-bone up to the right side of the tailbone.

    *Caution: Roll to the right side of your tailbone, then up that side. **Never** put your weight on the bottom tip of the tailbone.*

4. With your knees bent, both feet flat on the floor, and your hands on the floor behind you, move your body slightly forward and roll the ball a quarter inch up the right side of the sacrum, the flat, pear-shaped bone at the bottom of the spinal column. The ball should be pressing into bone, not muscle. Now, really concentrate on your breathing: inhale, and as you exhale sink your weight into the bone.

5. Continue to roll in micromovements up the right side of the sacrum. You are trying to stimulate the bone itself.

Tip for step 5

• *To get the most out of the back routine as a whole, take as much time as you can at your sacrum, sinking as deeply as you can into the ball. The sacrum is where the small muscles of your back begin, and stimulating these tiny muscles at this point sets off a release up the entire back. This stimulation will also improve bone quality and wake up the nerve roots.*

6. When the ball reaches the top of your sacrum, slowly roll it up off the sacrum and onto the right side of the bottom vertebra of your lower back. Inhale deeply, then exhale slowly, sinking your weight into the bone. Now, in micromovements, start to roll the ball slowly up the right side of your spine, taking a full breath at each movement as described in chapter 3 (page 53). Your feet push against the floor to help you move, while your hands help you balance. Your intention is to lift each vertebra away from the one below it and to stimulate and elongate the small muscles.

   Remember: *The ball should be pressing into the right side of the vertebrae all the way up the spine in order to release the tiny spinal muscles. Don't roll* across *the spine.*

Tips for step 6

- *You know you're at the top of the sacrum when you feel that you're at the top of your pelvic bone.*

- *Each deep inhalation lifts you slightly off the ball. Each exhalation deflates you so your body sinks heavily into the ball. You'll know when your muscles let go because on the exhalation, the body will sink deeper into the ball. At tight spots, you might want to stay for several breaths.*

7. As you roll slowly up the lower part of the right side of your spine, start to curve your buttocks down and around the ball. Meanwhile, as you inhale, feel your back expand out to where the ball is; as you exhale, sink down into the ball. Your buttocks are gradually dropping toward the floor.

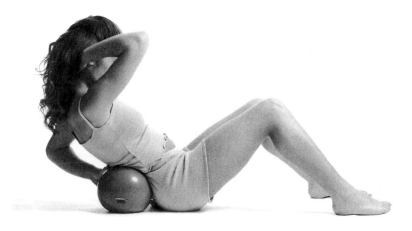

Step 8

8. When your buttocks reach the floor, the ball will be fully supporting the entire lower spine. Now raise your hands to gently support your head so it doesn't drop backward. If you feel you're losing balance, use one hand to push the ball into your lower back as the other hand supports your head and neck.

Tip for step 8

- *At no time should your head drop back unsupported. Use one hand to support your head, leaving the other hand free to keep you balanced.*

9. Sliding forward, continue to roll up your back, one inch at a time. At each point, exaggerate your inhale so you feel your back pressing out into the ball. At each exhale sink, sink, sink into the ball. At the *end* of each exhalation, slide the ball up the next inch. Continue until the ball is at shoulder level, pressing against the right side of the spine, between the spine and the shoulder blade.

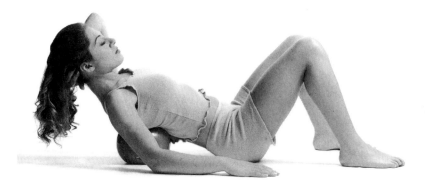

Step 9

Tip for step 9

- *As you roll, your abdominal muscles may begin to quiver, indicating that they need strengthening. As you continue doing this routine, they will indeed grow stronger, since Body Rolling offers powerful core strengthening and balance.*

10. Now pull your head all the way forward with your left hand. Bring your chin to your chest and roll the ball up into the right side of your neck. Let your neck and head come to rest against the ball. Your chin should remain pointed down toward your chest. Try to lower your right shoulder to the floor and pull it toward your feet. Your right palm faces the ceiling.

Tip for step 10

- *Pulling your chin toward your chest keeps the back of the neck elongated and straight on the ball. Don't turn your neck—turning prevents you from fully elongating your neck muscles.*

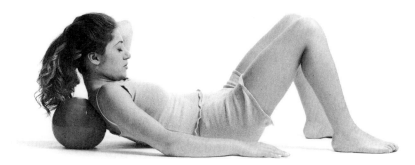

Step 10, chin to chest

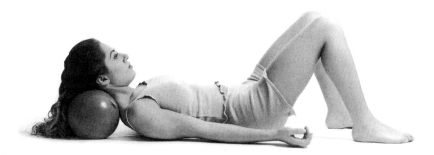

Step 10, head and neck resting around ball

11. Continue inhaling and exhaling. As you inhale, feel the right side of your neck pressing out into the ball; as you exhale, feel it sinking into the ball. Now return to micromovements, trying to move the ball in tiny increments up the back of your neck. Be sure to keep your head straight; don't turn it off to one side.

Tip for step 11

*   *If you can't keep your head straight, it's because your neck muscles are tight. As you continue doing this routine, those muscles will release.*

12. When the ball is just below your skull, feel it pushing up against the bony ridge at the bottom of your skull. Imagine that you're

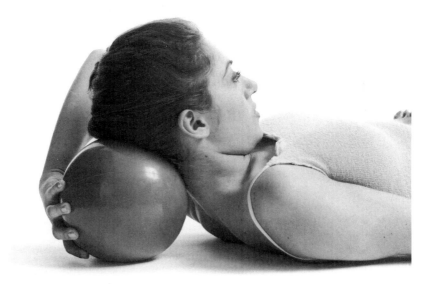

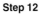
Step 12

separating your skull from your neck. Keep scooting forward; as you do the ball will roll up onto the right side of the back of the skull. Roll up to the very top of the back of your head, continuing to pull your right shoulder away from your head. Use your left hand to hold the ball so it doesn't pop out from under you.

13. To finish, support your neck with your right hand, roll the ball out from under you with your left hand, and use your right hand to slowly lower your head. Extend your legs out on the floor, arms alongside your body. Take a couple of deep breaths and notice any difference you feel between this side of your body and the left side.

14. If you have time, stand up and walk around, noticing the difference between the sides as you move.

15. Repeat the routine on the left side.

Lower Back Pain

If you have an occasional spasm in your lower back; acute lower back pain with inflammation, swelling, and heat; or a slipped or protruding disk in your lower back, I suggest starting with the following abdominal routine instead of the basic back routine. We frequently hear talk about how important the abdominal muscles are for a healthy back. This routine will release the psoas, an important abdominal muscle that attaches to the front side of the spine and is often so tight that it causes pain in the lower back. Working the abdomen will take the tension out of the psoas and the other abdominal muscles and elongate them, which by itself will often relieve pressure in the lower back and relax the lower back muscles. Constipation and the tendency to hold tension in the abdomen can also cause lower back pain, so this is another reason that the abdominal routine is the best place to begin correcting lower back discomfort.

If your back feels okay after you do the abdominal routine, you can then move on to the basic back routine.

Abdominal Routine for the Lower Back

Use a soft ball (equivalent to my yellow ball). If you only have a harder ball, deflate it a bit to make it softer.

1. Lie facedown with the ball pressing into your pubic bone (the bone between your legs at the bottom of the front of your pelvis). Your weight should be equally distributed on your knees, feet, and forearms so not all your weight is pressing into the ball.

2. Stay here for a minute or two, breathing and relaxing. Then slowly slide your body backward so the ball rolls partly up into your abdomen while still touching the top of the pubic bone. Each time the ball sinks deeper into the abdomen, curve your

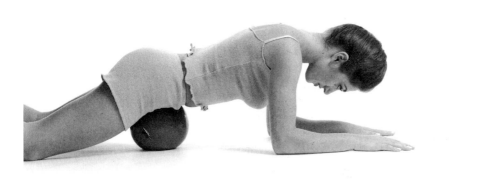

Step 1

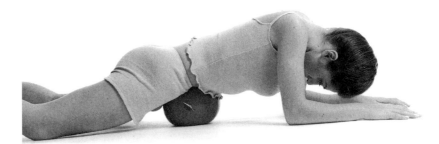

Step 2, pubic bone curving down around ball

pubic bone down around it toward the floor to take the ball in deeper toward the spine. You aren't moving the ball any farther toward the ribs—you want it to stay low in the abdomen. This routine isn't about moving the ball up to the ribs but about sinking deeper into the lower belly. Imagine you are pushing the ball toward your lower back.

Tip for step 2

- *The key to doing this routine successfully is the breathing. On the inhalation, your abdomen expands and pushes the ball out. The challenge comes with the exhale: letting yourself sink into the ball as*

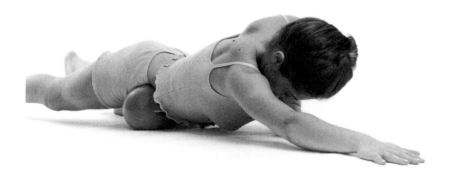

Step 3

much as possible. The moment you feel uncomfortable, you inhale, which releases the pressure. In this way you can use your breath to keep any discomfort at a level you can tolerate. (See the instructions for the abdominal routine on page 91 for more on this.)

3. Now move your body to the left, so the ball rolls into your right hip and pushes against that hip bone. Extend your right leg and arm out from your body as far as possible, inhale, and let the ball sink into your abdomen as you exhale.

Tip for step 3

- *This is an* active *stretch. You're working to achieve as much length as you can on your right side. As you stretch out your right arm and leg, you can feel how the abdominal muscles connect to both arm and leg. The more elongated the abdominals, the freer your arm and leg become.*

4. Roll the ball to the left hip and repeat step 3.

The Back Routine Against the Wall

This routine is good for people who find it hard to get down on the ground. You can do it almost anywhere that you have a wall and a ball. In this exercise, you aren't *rolling* the ball against the wall; rather, you're using your hands to move it from one point to the next. Because it involves pushing back against the wall, this routine also strengthens the core muscles and quadriceps (the front-of-thigh muscles). You may need to remove your shoes and socks so that your feet don't slide along the floor.

1. Standing with your back to the wall and your feet one to one and a half feet from the baseboard, place the ball as low as you can on the right side of your sacrum and lean back into it.

2. Now step away from the wall and use your hands to move the ball slightly up the right side of the sacrum, then lean back against the ball. Stay at this point for about 15 seconds, or longer if you like. Repeat about three times until the ball reaches the top of the sacrum.

3. When the ball reaches the right side of your lower back, begin using your breathing. Press back against the ball on the inhale, then sink into it on the exhale. You can also try using your hands to press the ball upward into each vertebra to get the sensation of creating space between the vertebrae. You'll feel a lift in the lower back.

4. Continue using your hands to move the ball up the right side of your spine until it's between your shoulder blades. Now press your body back into the ball, grip with your feet, and roll the ball out so it presses against your right shoulder blade, pushing the shoulder blade out to the side. Stay here for several breaths. This maneuver helps release the tension so many people develop between their shoulder blades.

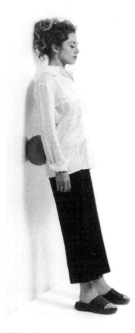

Step 1

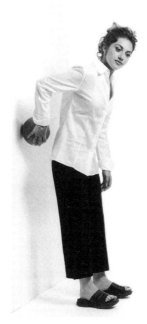

Step 2

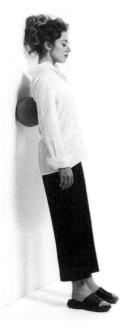

Step 4, ball moving up toward shoulder blades

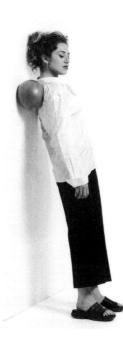

Step 4, ball pressing against shoulder blade

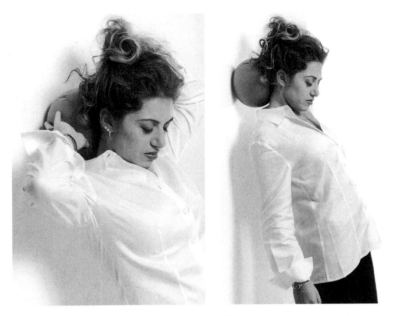

Step 6, pulling head forward   Step 6, pressing neck against ball

Tip for step 4

- *Since the back routine against the wall doesn't create as much length in your back as the floor version does, I've added this extra step, which helps release upper body tension by creating some extra width across your back.*

5. Bring the ball back to the right side of the spine and continue rolling up to shoulder level.

6. With your left hand, pull your head forward. With your right hand, move the ball up into your neck, lean back, and press your neck into it. Let go of your head and relax your arms down to your sides.

7. Shift your weight to the left so the ball rolls away from your spine, along the right side of the back of your neck. Roll out in small increments toward the bone behind your ear. You should be able to stop at two or three points before you reach the ear.

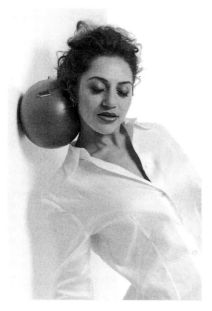

Step 7

As you roll, turn your body to the right so that when you reach the ear, your right side is facing the wall.

Tip for step 7

- *If you feel that the ball might pop out from behind your neck, use your left hand to hold it in place, gently guiding it toward the ear.*

8. Press your neck against the ball, then begin slowly turning to the left as you roll back to the spine in a continuous movement.

9. Repeat on the left side.

The Back Routine in a Chair

I find that whenever I'm stuck sitting somewhere for hours, I get more tired than if I were active. This routine lets you get the most out of those hours when you can't do anything but sit. I recommend doing this exercise at work, in an airplane, or on a train or bus. Instead of feeling stiff when you stand up, you're revitalized, since you've been working out the entire time you were sitting.

If you habitually sit for many hours, you can use the ball all day to continuously remind yourself to lean back. This will prevent you from becoming frozen in a slouched-forward posture.

1. Sitting in a chair, place the ball against the right side of your sacrum and lean back to press into it, keeping your back as straight as you can. Keep it there several seconds.

2. Using your hands, move the ball in small increments up the right side of your back, as far up as the chair back allows. Keep the ball at each point for several seconds as you lean back against it.

3. Repeat on the left side.

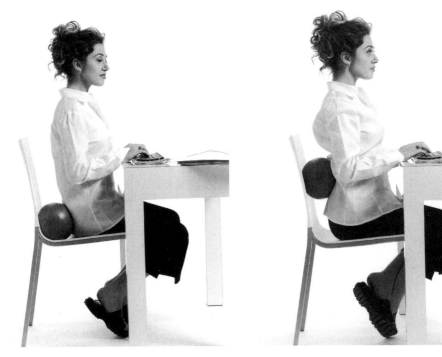

Step 1   Step 2

5

The Pelvis: Hips, Abdomen, and Buttocks

Everyone wants the flat belly or "buns of steel" that will make them look sexy and feel great. We often work hard to achieve that toned, tight look. But now you no longer need to put forth all that effort. Body Rolling will give you the flat abdomen, toned buttocks, and sleek hips you dream of, easier and faster than any other type of workout.

Many fitness regimes target just the hips or abdomen or buttocks. But treating these areas in isolation won't produce the desired results, for they're actually all components of one important structure: the pelvis.

One way or another, we all focus on the pelvis as a gauge of how we look and feel. Women are likely to put on weight around their pelvis, then worry about how to make this area slimmer and more attractive. Men, for their part, try to live up to our society's blueprint for physical manliness and sex appeal, making their bodies as tight and hard as they can. This leads to the classic "Marlboro Man" posture, with the pelvis thrust forward and the buttocks very tense and clenched. Although aesthetically desirable, over time this posture can actually cause lower back pain and even shoulder and neck problems.

For men and women both, the mainstream fitness dogma of tightening the pelvic area will ultimately do little to help you achieve the shape you want. And because you're tightening the area, rather than freeing it, you invite a host of body architecture problems. Body Rolling, by contrast, will streamline your pelvis by releasing all its muscles, even as it tones them.

The Architecture of the Pelvis

I see the pelvis as a single entity, not a separate front, back, and sides. It's a fundamental part of your architecture, for it takes more stress than any other part of the body. When you walk, your feet transmit pressure up into the pelvis, while your upper body bears weight down into it from above. In fact, every time you sit or stand, you're using muscles attached to the pelvis. The pelvis therefore has to be the stablest, strongest structure in the body. Its strength and integrity hold you up and prevent many structural problems. The strong muscles you have on all sides of it are designed for just this purpose.

All the thigh muscles attach to the pelvic bone, so to give the pelvis its full range of motion, you need toned, elongated thigh muscles. The abdominal and back muscles attach the ribs to the pelvis, and these muscles must be able to support the upper body so it doesn't give in to gravity and drop down, putting stress into the pelvis. Even the gluteal muscles, or buttocks, have an important structural function. People tend to think of their buttocks purely in aesthetic terms, but in fact, the gluteal muscles' job is to separate the back from the legs. They help prevent the torso from exerting extra pressure down into the lower back and prevent the legs from exerting upward pressure into the pelvis. Not only do all the pelvic muscles need to be long and strong; they must also be balanced—that is, of equal length and strength on all sides.

One reason Body Rolling is so effective is that it targets the pelvis as a whole, instead of focusing on specific parts. If your pelvic muscles are tight in general, your legs won't move freely, and your back and abdominal muscles will be pulled downward, restricting the movement of your torso. The result is a short-waisted body with "love handles," legs that look as though they're jammed up into the pelvis, and thick upper thighs.

This chapter gives you five routines for releasing the front, back, and sides of the pelvis; restoring its balance; and creating a longer, leaner, and more flexible torso, as well as freer movement in the legs and hips. If you do these routines, you'll also find that your hips and thighs begin to look longer and more slender, and that your buttocks achieve the kind of firmness you desire.

Creating Space for Organs

All our internal organs are encased within our rib cage and pelvis. These organs function better when there's plenty of space inside the rib cage and between the rib cage and the pelvis. This space ensures that they receive adequate blood circulation. But due to our sedentary lifestyle, the effects of gravity, and poor posture, most people's upper body slowly collapses down into the pelvis, compressing the organs, pushing them down out of their proper places, and slowing their function.

In a large, collapsed belly, for example, the muscles have no tone and organ function decreases. There is excess downward pressure on the intestines, which slows digestion, since there is less space for peristalsis, the waves of contraction that move the digesting food through the intestinal tract. The person becomes bloated and finds it impossible to lose weight because his or her organ function is so depressed. Dropped intestines also exert pressure on the bladder, often leading (especially for women who have had children) to a dropped (prolapsed) bladder; and they cut off circulation in the legs, causing varicose veins.

An article of faith among fitness buffs is that to have a strong back, you need strong abdominal muscles. This is one reason for doing crunches and sit-ups. But crunches contract, tighten, and harden the abdominal area, thus shortening the space between the rib cage and the pelvis. This not only decreases space for the vital organs, but causes just those lower back problems that the exercisers hope to avoid. When you shorten the space in the torso, you also shorten the spine, diminishing the spaces between the vertebrae—and leading to a different kind of "crunch" in the lower back. So your abdominal muscles need to be not just tight and strong, but also as long as possible. Elongating tight abdominal muscles with Body Rolling and using the ball to retrain these muscles to hold up the torso creates more space for your organs and keeps them in their proper place.

Sitting Awareness

The main reason so many of us have weak abdominal muscles is that we spend all day sitting. No one teaches us that how we sit affects the health of our internal organs by decreasing the space available for them. So one thing you can do to firm your belly and enhance the health of your internal organs is to change the way you sit. If you engage your abdominals during the day, rather than just letting them hang, they'll become toned and keep your organs from dropping. Try this little exercise:

- Put your hand on your belly and inhale. As you exhale, consciously pull your abdominal muscles in toward the center of your body. Feel the inward movement with your hand.

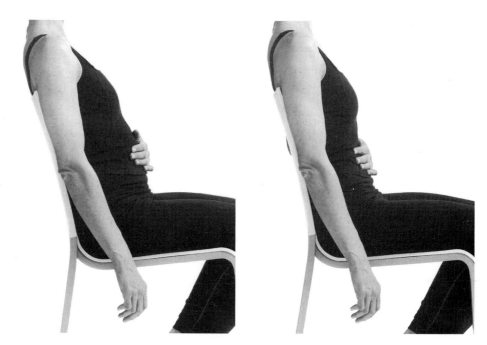

Inhale

Exhale

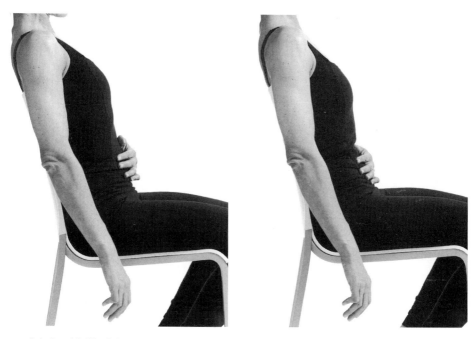

Inhale with lifted rib cage

Exhale with lifted rib cage

- Relax your shoulders down, and keep them relaxed as you do this exercise. With your hand still on your belly, inhale again, this time lifting your rib cage so that the air goes into your chest. This lift elongates the abdominal muscles, creating space between your abdomen and rib cage and allowing the abdominals to move slightly inward. As you exhale, keep your rib cage lifted, feeling the abdominals move still further inward. This upright posture, with long abdominals, is your optimal sitting position.

Naturally no one can remember to sit like this every moment of the day. But if you remind yourself to return to this posture periodically—even while you sit at your desk and work—it can turn into a habit. Over time it will give you the strong, lean abdominals you want.

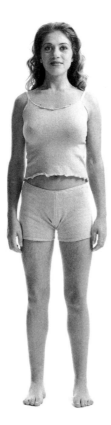

Optimal pelvis alignment

Optimal Pelvis Alignment

- Both hips are the same height.

- Your pelvis is centered, not tilted forward or backward.

- At least two inches separate the bottom of the rib cage from the top of the hip bone.

Self-Exam

- First, notice where your two hip bones are. Are they the same height? You can tell by observing whether the waistline of your pants falls differently from one side to the other.

- Are your hips rotated so that one is forward and one is backward? To find out, hook your thumbs around your hips and feel whether they're in the same position.

- Are both hips rotated forward? This tilts the pelvis forward, making the buttocks stick out and forcing the lower back into a swayback.

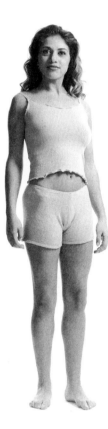

One hip rotated forward, one backward

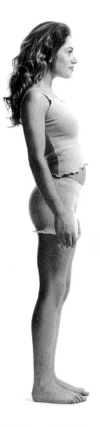

Both hips rotated forward

- Are both hips rotated backward? This tilts the pelvis backward, so the tailbone is tucked under. The back is flat, with no curve, the pubic bone comes forward, and the buttocks muscles either collapse and sag or grip tightly (in men, this tight grip creates the classic "Marlboro Man" posture).

- Look at your legs. Are your feet and legs facing forward or turned out? If they turn out, your hip movement will be restricted.

- Can you turn both legs in and out equally? This movement depends on muscles called rotators that attach the lower part

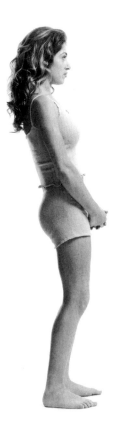

Both hips rotated backward

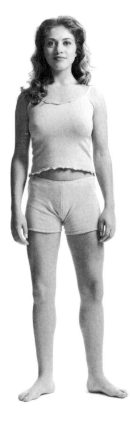

Legs turned out

of the pelvic bone to the upper thighbone. If the rotators are contracted, they limit leg and hip movement.

- Look at your buttocks. Are they dropped and sagging, or toned and solid? If they're sagging, they're not supporting your pelvis.

- Look at your abdomen. Does it drop over your pelvis, or is it uplifted, holding your torso erect? Try taking it in your hands and lifting it up. If you can lift it, it's dropped.

Hamstring Release

The first step in working on your pelvis is the hamstring release, which tones and elongates the muscles in the backs of your thighs, helping to free your gluteal muscles.

1. Place the ball under your right sitbone, sinking all your weight into it (for instructions on finding your sitbone, see page 49). Use your hands or fingertips on the floor to help support you

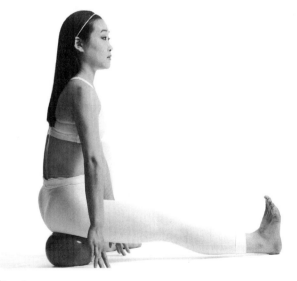

Step 1

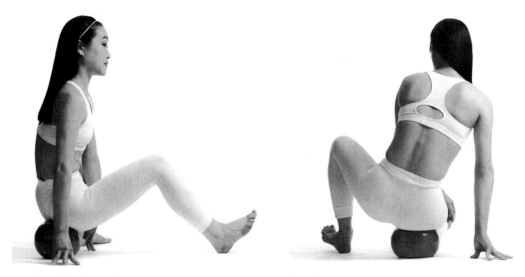

Step 2, rolling forward

Step 3

and for balance. Your right leg extends straight out in front of you; the left leg is bent, with your left foot flat on the floor. The left leg also helps you balance and move on the ball. Your right leg will bend a bit as you move the ball around the sitbone.

2. Use your fingertips and left foot to gently move your body forward and backward so the ball rolls behind, then in front of, the sitbone.

3. Now shift your body weight from side to side on the ball, building up momentum so the ball rolls from one end of the right sitbone to the other end.

4. Roll clockwise and counterclockwise around the right sitbone.

5. Using your fingertips and left foot, pull your body backward and roll the ball a couple of inches down the back of your right leg. Take a full breath in and, as you exhale, let the back of the leg sink into the ball, elongating the hamstrings.

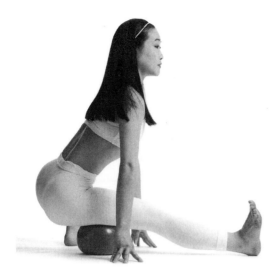

Step 5

6. Continue to roll in two-inch increments, sinking and waiting at each point, about two-thirds of the way to your knee.

7. Repeat on the left side.

Buttocks Lifter

I always give this exercise to classes of women, and they're amazed at how their buttocks perk up so quickly. I call this the "butt-lifter." If you want a new shape to your derrière, it's a must for your workout.

Since most of us don't really use our gluteal muscles, they tend to sag instead of performing their function of holding up the pelvis. As a result, the back of the pelvis drops, putting pressure into the legs and lower back and creating a drooping look. This routine will wake up the gluteal muscles so they start to function as they should. It's also excellent for releasing tight hips.

1. Place the ball just below your right sitbone, at the point where the hamstring muscles attach to this bone. Your right knee is

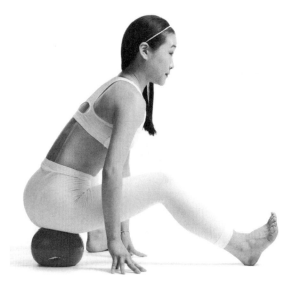

Step 1

slightly bent, your fingertips are on the floor in front of you, and your torso leans forward. Your left leg is bent, with the foot flat on the floor.

2. Pull your torso forward so that your chest comes toward your knee. Let your weight bear down onto the ball. Now sit up straight as you roll the ball back up onto your sitbone.

3. Extend your body straight up as you let your weight bear straight down into the ball. Bring your hands behind you for balance and start to roll up your buttock in small increments, bearing down with all your weight into the ball. The ball lifts your buttock as you roll. Roll about halfway to the top of the pelvic bone, then bring the ball back to the starting position just below your sitbone.

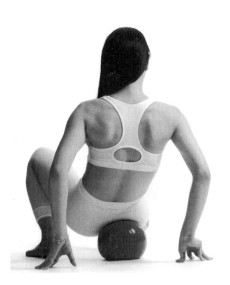

Step 3

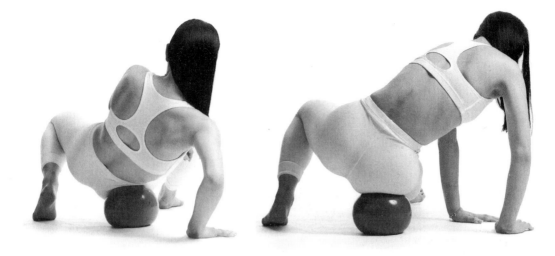

Step 4

Step 5, rolling to edge of sitbone

4. Roll up onto your sitbone again. Now roll the ball outward, in the direction of the right shoulder. You're not rolling up the outside of the hip, but up the right side of your right buttock. As you roll, shift additional weight onto your left foot. Your torso leans to the right, supported on your right hand. Roll about two-thirds of the way toward the top of the pelvic bone, then return again to the starting position below your sitbone.

> As you do this routine, bear down with all your weight onto the ball as you roll up onto the sitbone, so the ball can push the gluteal muscle up. This action is what provides the lift.

5. Now bring both hands to your right side, lean your body to the right, and roll up onto the sitbone. Roll in small increments—as tiny as you can manage—sideways out to the right edge of the sitbone, then trace a half-circle up around the outside of your thigh and hip, ending at the point where the thigh bone meets the pelvis.

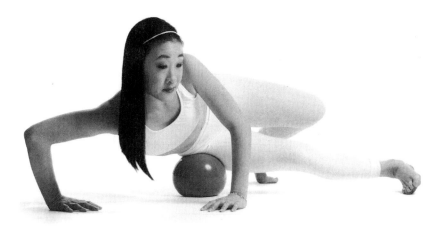

Step 5, tracing a half-circle around the thigh

6. Roll off the ball.

7. Repeat on the left side.

Working the Abdomen

More than anywhere else in the body, working with the ball in the abdomen is a challenge, since all the pressure is directed into muscles and organs, not into bone. You can sink deeper here than elsewhere, but the sensation can be intense.

I tell all my students that when they first do this routine, their minds might panic and say, "This can't be good for me!" "This is crazy!" "This will hurt my intestines!" and so on. I reassure them that it won't. We rarely massage our intestinal area, but Body Rolling gives you a way to go in as deep as is comfortable for you and begin to stimulate this area, releasing tension, increasing circulation and peristalsis, and breaking up old scar tissue—both on the surface of the body and internally. Most of us grow sluggish and congested in our abdomen, and it's important to understand that there's a healthy way to stimulate it physically to tone the organs and muscles. So use your mind to counteract your anxiety. Tell yourself, "This is okay! I'm only going as far as I feel comfortable. It's safe." And remind yourself that, above all, this exercise is a great way to flatten your belly.

Nevertheless, keep in mind that although the sensation may be intense, you're not supposed to subject yourself to pain. The trick is to use your breathing to control how deep you go. As you inhale, push against the ball, as though you were pushing it out of your abdomen. Then as you exhale, control the amount of air you release, so you sink into the ball only as much as you can tolerate. During the sink you can feel tightness and tension in your abdomen, but with each breath, the discomfort will melt away a bit more. The ball might be at a point that feels quite hard, but on the next breath, the area will begin to soften, and you'll be able to let the ball in a little deeper. Since we're usually not aware of how much tension we hold in our bellies, you're likely to find this routine quite enlightening.

Front Hip Release

You can't imagine what this release feels like until you do it. To get the full effect, be sure to wait the full 30 seconds in step 1, and don't forget the twist in step 3.

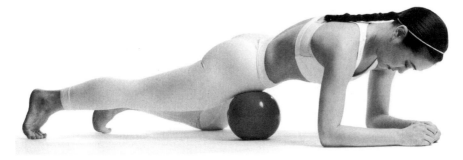

1. Lying facedown, place the ball directly on the part of the right hipbone that touches the floor. The ball is on bone, not muscle. Try not to drop the left hip; your hips should be parallel to the floor. Your right leg is extended, and your weight rests on your forearms, left knee and foot, and right toes. Stay here, with the ball pressing into the bone, for at least 30 seconds, breathing and sinking. This wait stimulates the bone and the muscle tendons attached to it to let go.

2. Shift your weight to the right. This is a tiny movement—a microshift. The ball will slide off the bone into the abdomen, but it still hugs the inside curve of the hip. Extend that right leg out nice and long with your toes on the floor but your knee off the floor, walk your right arm out long on the floor past your head, and take two or three deep breaths, letting the ball sink in.

3. Now cross your right forearm in front of you on the floor for support. Your left palm presses into the floor at shoulder level. Twist your torso upward to the left. Each time you exhale, the right side of your hip slides down toward the floor so that your

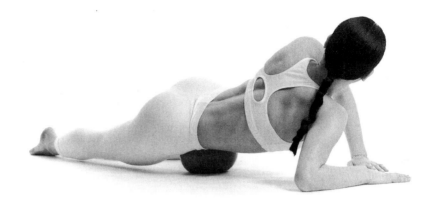

hip is almost falling off the ball. This moves the ball toward the center of your abdomen. Stay here for about four deep breaths, twisting your torso and head farther to the left with each breath.

Tip for Step 3

- *The ball itself does not move. As you breathe and sink, you're sliding around it. With each breath, the ball can sink deeper into the abdomen.*

4. Repeat on the left side.

Core Toning and Release

The sensation this routine produces is quite intense, but the results are amazing: a flatter belly and flatter back. What's more, the routine repositions your center of gravity, taking pressure off your lower back, so you'll find yourself standing with far greater ease.

1. Lying facedown, place the ball at the center of your pubic bone. Resting on your knees and forearms, stay here for 30 seconds, breathing and sinking.

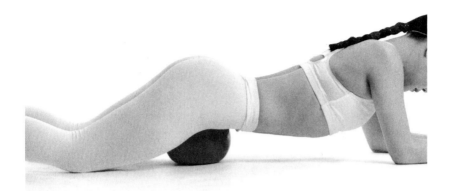

Step 1

Tips for step 1

- *Here again, you begin by stimulating bone. At the same time, you're releasing tension in your sacrum, since pressing into the pubic bone relaxes the entire pelvis.*

- *Resting the ball on your pubic bone should not be painful. Sometimes, for example if you're premenstrual, the bone might feel tender. But if it's always sensitive, consult your doctor.*

2. Shift your weight to the left and roll the ball in a micromovement to the right side of the pubic bone. Stay here for 10 seconds.

3. Shift your weight to the right and roll the ball in a micromovement to the left side of the pubic bone. Stay here for 10 seconds.

4. Bring the ball back to center. Slowly slide your body backward so the ball rolls to the top of the pubic bone and begins to sink into the abdomen. The ball should be partly on the pubic bone and partly pressing into your abdomen.

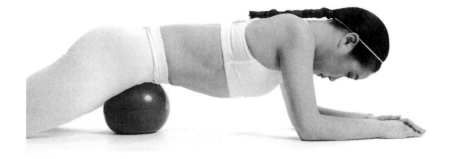

Step 5

Tip for step 4

- *This is the point where the longest abdominal muscle attaches to the pubic bone. From here this muscle runs straight up to the breastbone and rib cage. After years of bad posture and hours of sitting, this muscle starts to sag and loses its function of holding the body erect. What you're doing now is stimulating it to regain that function.*

5. Tighten your buttocks and push your pubic bone down around the ball toward the floor, so it curves around the ball. As you breathe, the ball sinks deeper into the abdomen. The breathing creates a release that moves the ball up toward your navel.

Tips for step 5

- *You're not moving your body; it's the extra length in the muscle that gives the ball space to move.*

- *Your buttocks should not stick up in the air. Work toward a flat lower back, with your buttocks pushing down toward the floor.*

6. When the ball reaches the level of your navel, extend your legs, lifting your knees so that just your toes are on the floor. Extend

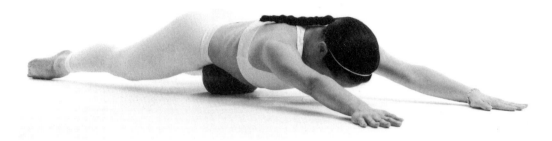

Step 6

your arms above your head, walking your fingertips along the floor in front of you. Breathe deeply, letting the ball sink into your abdomen. Take three full breaths, exaggerating the inhalation and sinking in as deeply as you can on the exhalation, in order to get the full benefit. At the same time, work to stretch your arms and legs out as long as you can, concentrating on creating as much length as possible in the torso.

Tip for step 6

- *The exhalation is a real challenge; you're intensely stimulating all your internal organs. Often there is gas, tension, or constipation in the intestines that makes lying over the ball painful. If the sensation is too intense, inhale to relieve the discomfort.*

7. Get off the ball. Lie on your back and feel how much flatter your lower back is on the floor.

Sciatica Routine

One type of sciatica is due to tight muscles in the buttocks and thighs that press into the sciatic nerve, causing pain that shoots down the leg. The following routine will help relieve this type of sciatica. However, it may not help the second form of sciatica, which is caused by compression in the lower back that irritates a nerve root. If this routine fails to relieve your pain, try the abdominal routine on pages 69–71. If neither routine is effective, consult a health-care professional. As long as pain from sciatica persists, avoid the basic back routine.

1. Lean back and place the ball at the top of your right hipbone, touching the right side of your spine. Your weight should be distributed equally on your feet, hip, and hands. Your hands are on the floor behind you.

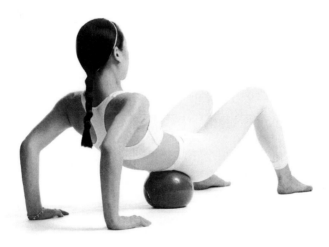

Step 1

2. Now shift more weight onto your left arm. Roll the ball just below the top of the hipbone, then roll it out toward the right, angling down toward the point where the right thighbone goes

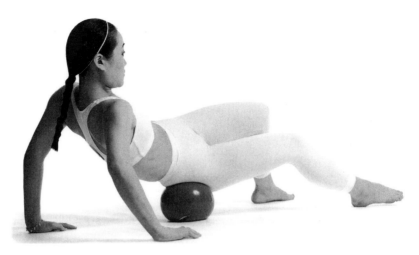

Step 2

into the pelvis (the hip joint). Roll slowly out toward this point, breathing and sinking at each point, until the ball reaches the hip joint.

3. Bring the ball back to the starting position, then roll down an inch, so the ball is on the upper part of your sacrum. Stay here, sink, and breathe. Shift your weight to the left again and roll sideways down to the right hip joint, sinking and breathing at each point.

4. Bring the ball back to the starting position, roll it an inch farther down the sacrum, and roll out to the hip joint again.

5. Bring the ball back to the starting position once more and roll it another inch farther down until it's close to your tailbone. Now roll the ball to the right, out to the hip joint.

6. Repeat on the left side.

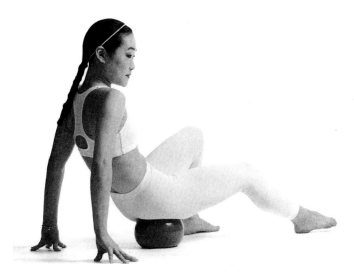

Step 5, ball near tailbone

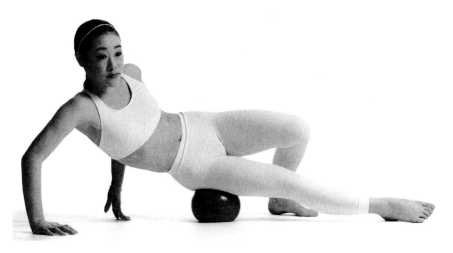

Step 5, rolling out to hip joint

6

Legs

How much attention do you pay to the way you walk? Most of us don't think about walking at all. From the moment we find our balance as babies, we just get up on our feet and take off. No one teaches us how to walk, and we don't give our leg function much thought as long as we can get where we want to go. Athletes working toward peak performance learn from a trainer to use their legs optimally. Dancers, yoga students, and martial artists are trained in how to stand. But the rest of us just go with whatever we've got.

At the same time, most of us do focus a lot on how our legs *look*. Women usually yearn for long, lean, toned, well-proportioned legs, while men want strong legs with well-defined muscles. But even though you work out hard, using a Stairmaster or doing step aerobics, you may still not be getting the look you want. That's because, unless your leg muscles are properly aligned—which means balanced, flexible, and free-moving—you won't be able to change their shape.

People who exercise have an additional reason to pay attention to their leg alignment. Their legs receive constant stress from the pressure exerted by the rest of the body during the workout. Most cardiovascular exercise involves repetitive leg movements. Doing these movements with legs that aren't well aligned may lead to a knee, ankle, or hip injury. Doing lower body strengthening workouts—squats or deep knee bends, machines or weights—without good alignment can also cause injuries.

Whatever your leg alignment patterns, you walk with them every day, so it's worth developing an awareness of them. In the following sections you'll discover what your patterns are, then use the Body Rolling leg routines to balance your legs by freeing all these muscles and elongating them so that they're all the same length. These leg routines will correct any misalignments you may have. Better yet—unlike other fitness practices that bulk up your thighs—Body Rolling will give you the improved shape you're after, by lengthening and streamlining your leg muscles.

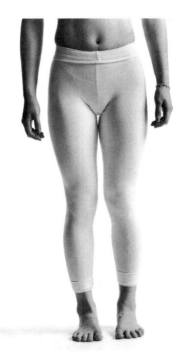

Optimal leg alignment

Optimal Leg Alignment

The key to a solid leg structure that lets you do most activities injury-free is correct alignment of the thigh muscles and thighbone. The thighbone, the biggest bone in the body, connects the legs to the pelvis. Three muscle groups attach to the thighbone: the hamstrings in back, the quadriceps in the front, and the adductors in the inner thigh. To keep that bone properly aligned in the hip socket, all three muscle groups must be flexible, toned, and balanced—which means equally elongated and fully performing their function.

Along the outside of the thigh runs a powerful band of connective tissue to which the hamstrings and quadriceps attach. Often these muscles get stuck to this connective tissue, unbalancing the leg.

In optimally aligned legs

- Both thighbones descend straight down from the hips.

- The knees face directly forward.

- Both shins are straight, not turned in or out.

- The feet are directly under your hips and point straight forward.

Self-Exam

First, think about daily habits that may affect your legs. Ask yourself these questions:

- Do you tend to stand on one leg more than the other?

- Do you always cross the same leg over the other when you sit?

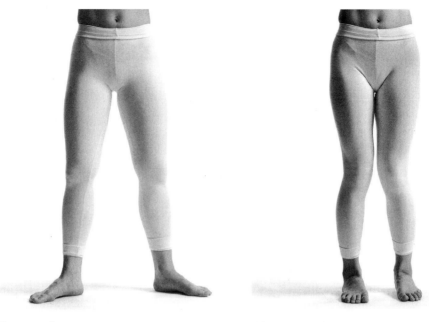

Feet turned out   **Thighs rotated inward**

- Do you play tennis or another one-sided sport? This means that you're putting more pressure on one leg than on the other.

Now, observe your legs in the mirror.

- Are your feet turned out?

- Are your legs wider apart than your hips?

- Do your thighs rotate inward? Notice whether your thigh muscles seem pulled toward the inner thigh.

- Do your knees face straight forward or are they turned inward (knock-knees) or outward?

- Now turn sideways and look at your calf. Is it in a straight line with your thigh or is the calf actually behind the thigh? If it is, your knee is hyperextended.

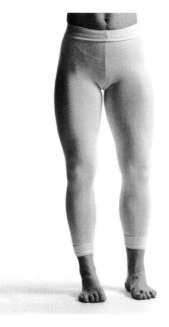

Knees turned out

- Face forward again. Is there a general thickness around your knees? This thickness can have two causes. The first is contracted thigh muscles. The second is extra weight in the thighs, which exerts additional pressure into the knees. If you have that extra weight, on top of any of the misalignments noted above, you may be more likely to injure your knees because of additional wear and tear on the joint.

Doing the leg routines will confirm the existence of any misalignments you saw in the mirror, since you'll feel the corresponding tight muscles that cause these posture patterns.

How the Leg Routines Work

The routines that follow work the muscle groups of the thigh. Freeing, lengthening, and toning the thigh muscles will release the calf muscles as well. After doing these routines, you'll feel greater ease in walking and will develop greater range of motion and shock absorption in your knees, ankles, and hips. Athletes will see their running, jogging, and cycling improve. And doing the leg routines before or after any type of workout is a great way to prevent injury as well as improve performance.

These routines also break up cellulite, which consists of fatty deposits under the skin that develop in the parts of the body where movement is restricted because of short, contracted muscles or lack of muscle tone. The tissue becomes stagnant and congested: blood circulation and muscle tone decrease, the skin sags, and cellulite forms. This is often the case with women who gain their weight in their hips and thighs. You can't get rid of cellulite just by doing exercises to burn fat, because that won't realign and tone the individual muscles. You need to physically stimulate the area, rolling through the tissue, to get the circulation moving again. As you roll, the pressure of the ball breaks up the fatty deposits under the skin and tones the muscle.

In these routines, you roll only two-thirds of the way to the knee. That's because when the knee is extended, rolling all the way to the joint can injure the knee if you have a misalignment.

Toning the Hamstrings

Each thigh has three hamstring muscles. Two attach at the inner knee, and the third attaches at the outer knee. Step 6 works the whole muscle group; steps 7 and 8 work the outer hamstring; and steps 9 and 10 work the two inner ones.

As you roll down the muscles, you should feel the weight of your body pressing down into the ball, which at the same time exerts pressure up into the leg muscles. This routine actually irons out the hamstring muscles, which you'll experience as a sensation that the muscles are stretching out. You might not feel the full effect of rolling down your leg until you get off the ball, stand up and walk around. It's then that you will really see and feel the changes.

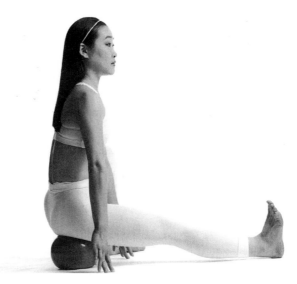

Step 1

1. Place the ball under your right sitbone, sinking all your weight into it. Use your hands or fingertips on the floor to help support you and for balance. Your right leg extends straight out in front of you; the left leg is bent, with your left foot flat on the floor. The left leg helps you balance and move on the ball. Your right leg will bend a bit as you move the ball around the sitbone.

2. Gently move your body forward and backward so the ball rolls behind, then in front of, the sitbone. Use your fingertips and left foot to shift yourself forward and backward.

3. Now shift your body weight from side to side on the ball, building up momentum so the ball rolls from one end of the right sitbone to the other end.

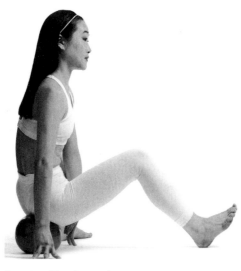

Step 2, rolling forward

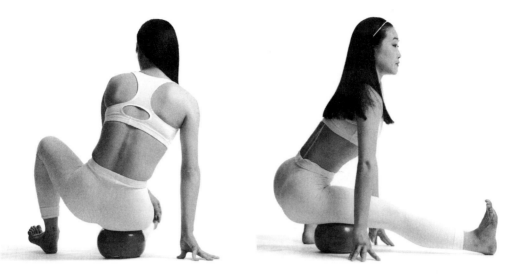

Step 3   Steps 5 and 6

4. Roll clockwise and counterclockwise around the right sitbone.

5. Now, using your fingertips and left foot, pull your body backward and roll the ball a couple of inches down the back of your right leg. Take a full breath in and as you exhale, let the back of the leg sink into the ball, stretching the hamstrings.

6. Continue to roll the ball forward in two-inch increments, sinking and waiting at each point, to about two-thirds of the way to your knee. Then roll the ball back up over the hamstring muscles to the sitbone in one smooth movement.

> If you can't roll the ball back up over your hamstrings, use your hands to take the ball out from under your leg and place it back under your sitbone.

7. Now roll the ball forward off the sitbone and shift your weight to the left, so the ball rolls to the right side of the back of your leg just below the sitbone. Place both your hands on the floor on your right side. Lean on your hands for support as you turn the leg out to the right.

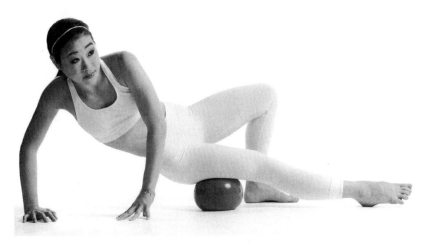

Step 8

8. Pull your body backward and roll the ball a couple of inches down the right leg, leaning to the right side so you're putting more weight into the outer hamstring muscle. The ball is rolling down the outside of the back of your thigh. Continue rolling in two-inch increments, to about two-thirds of the way to your knee.

Tip for step 8

• *Don't turn all the way onto your side here; if you do, you won't be on the hamstring anymore.*

9. Roll the ball back up to the sitbone as you straighten upward. Now keep the weight of your body between your legs and place your hands on the floor in front of you, between your legs.

10. Roll the ball off the sitbone, turn your right leg inward, and slide the ball slightly to the left, to the inside of the back of your thigh. The ball is now on your inner hamstring. Keep

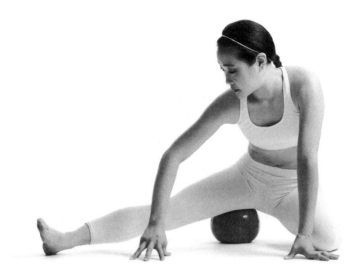

Steps 9 and 10

your leg turned inward as you bring your left knee down to the floor and turn it out slightly to the left. Then roll toward the right knee in two-inch increments as before.

Tip for step 10

- *If it's difficult to feel the two inner hamstring muscles, turn your left knee out a little farther to the left. You can also try leaning your torso more to the left as you bend forward.*

11. Repeat the entire routine on the left side.

Toning the Outside Thigh

It's common for the outside line of the thigh to be extremely tight, so don't be surprised if the sensation you feel during this routine is quite intense at first. This is what people often call a "good pain," because you know that it's basically beneficial. As you continue to do the exercise, it will become much easier.

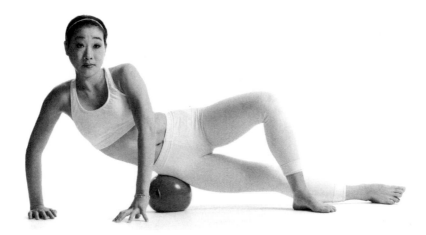

Step 1

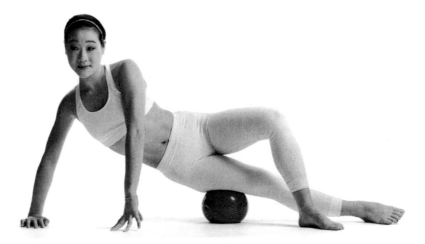

Step 2

1. Lying on your right side, place the ball at the point where your thighbone goes into your hip. Hold it there for about 30 seconds, letting all your weight drop into the ball. Your right hand supports your body. Your left hand is on the floor in front of you for balance. Your left foot is either in front of the right leg or behind it, depending on which position helps you balance more easily. Your right leg extends straight out.

2. Using both hands to pull your body in the direction of your head, roll the ball down the side of your leg about two inches. Stay here, breathing, for about 10 seconds.

3. Continue rolling down the leg in two-inch increments, holding for 10 seconds at each point. Roll about two-thirds of the way to the knee.

4. Repeat on the left side.

Tip for the outside thigh routine

- *This routine requires considerable arm strength (which doing the routine will develop). If it's too hard at first to hold your body up on a straight right arm, come down on your forearm.*

Toning the Front of the Thigh (Quadriceps)

Your quadriceps actually include five different muscles, which are usually stuck to each other and to the bone. Unlike hamstring tightness, which we easily feel when we bend over, it's hard to feel quad tightness in daily life, so we often don't realize how tight and out of shape our quads are until we do this routine. Because these muscles are generally so tight and restricted, this routine tends to be very challenging at first. However if you persevere, the intensity will subside. What's more, very soon you can usually feel and see the five muscles separating from each other as their individual definition emerges. Once your quads are released, you'll feel much more freedom in your legs, and you'll be surprised at how much easier it is to stand up straight.

1. Lie facedown and place the ball directly on the part of the right hipbone that touches the floor. Your right leg extends out behind you as you support yourself on your forearms, left knee, and right foot.

2. Pull your body forward, rolling the ball about five inches down so you feel it pressing into the thighbone itself. Keep your lower back straight as you let the weight of your leg sink into the ball.

Tips for step 2

- *Make sure you roll at least five inches down the leg, so that the ball is pressing into your thighbone, not your groin.*

- *Keep your abdominal muscles pulled in toward your spine, and keep your lower back flat. If you drop your belly you'll be in a swayback position and can hurt your lower back.*

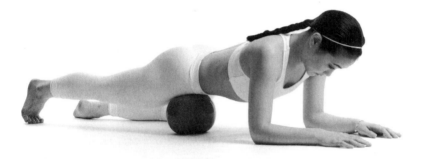

Step 1

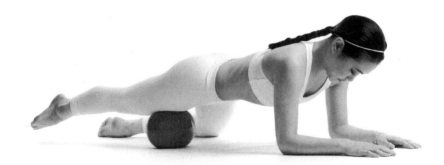

Step 2

3. Now slowly turn the leg out, keeping the knee straight, as you let the inner side of the quadriceps sink into the ball. It's important here to take the time to let the ball penetrate the muscle as deeply as possible.

4. Rotate the leg slowly back to center.

5. Next move your right forearm so it's in front of you, and move your left hand out to the side at shoulder level to support you. Slowly turn your torso to the left. This rolls the ball to the outside of the right leg. Stay here, wait, and sink, letting all the weight of your leg drop into the ball.

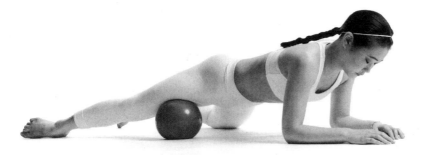

Step 3

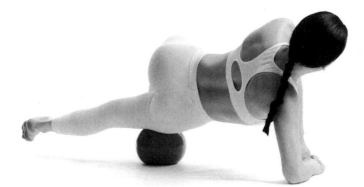

Step 5

6. Rotate slowly back to center, feeling the ball cross the quadriceps muscles.

Tip for steps 3–6

- *As the ball rolls over the quadriceps muscles, you'll feel a series of thunks as it crosses these muscles one after the other.*

7. Now pull your body forward another couple of inches. Repeat the roll to left and right in steps 3 to 6.

8. Repeat this roll at about three more points, ending about two-thirds of the way down the thigh.

9. Repeat on the left side.

Toning the Inner Thigh

Your adductor muscles lie between your quadriceps and hamstrings. Their job is to establish the balance between the front and back muscle groups that is essential to keep the leg aligned. Since most people don't realize how important the adductors are, this muscle group tends to be the "forgotten" muscle group of the leg. Dancers, yoga practitioners, and martial artists deliberately work these muscles, but in fitness routines and most daily activities people have no awareness of them. As a result these muscles are often unused and become atrophied. The quads and hamstrings then start to pull in toward the atrophied adductors, with the result that all these muscles get stuck together, which restricts them from fully performing their jobs.

If you have difficulty spreading your legs, crossing one ankle over the opposite knee, or sitting cross-legged, these muscles are probably the ones you need to work on. And, if you've been seeing any sagging or crinkly skin in your upper inner thighs or around your inner knees, this routine will tighten and tone it away.

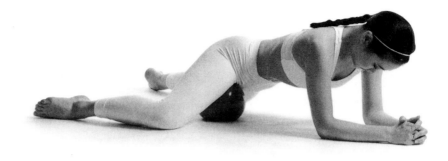

Step 1

1. Lie facedown, supporting yourself on your forearms. Bend your right knee and bring it up to hip level; it's very important to have the knee just at hip level, not above or below. Your left leg is extended straight out behind you. Now take the ball in your hand and place it at the point where the right inner thigh meets the pelvis (the groin). As you do this, your hips will lift off the floor; be sure to keep them level with each other. *You should not be lying on your left side.* Try to keep both hips the same distance from the floor (that is, try not to drop the left hip) as you let all your body weight sink into the ball. Remain here for about a minute, breathing and sinking.

Tips for step 1

- *To avoid lower back injury, it's essential to keep your abdominal muscles pulled in toward the spine and your lower back flat.*

- *If, like most people's, your adductors are atrophied, you might not feel the ball pressing into them. So it's important to remain with the ball pressing into your groin for a good 60 seconds, to wake these muscles up.*

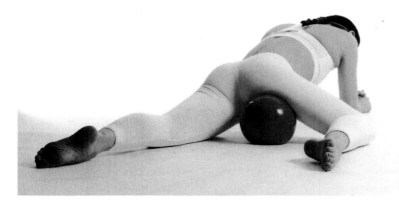

Step 2, ball rolling toward back of thigh

- *Keeping the left hip raised is challenging, so if you get tired, you can lower it to the floor. But continue working to keep your hips parallel to the floor, because this will increase the benefits of the routine.*

2. Now slide your body to the left so that the ball rolls along your inner thigh about two inches toward your knee. Microshift your body forward, so the ball rolls slightly toward the back of your thigh, and stay here for 30 seconds.

3. Now shift a bit backward, so the ball rolls slightly toward the front of your thigh, and wait again for 30 seconds.

4. Keep rolling in increments of two inches until the ball reaches your knee, shifting forward and backward at each point as in steps 2 and 3. Once the ball reaches the knee, you can lower your left hip to the floor.

Tip for step 4
- *When the leg is bent, it's safe to roll the ball all the way out to the knee.*

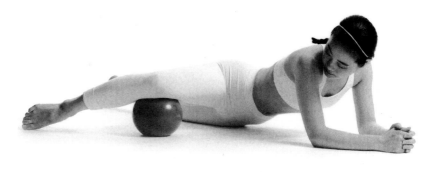

Step 4

5. Make small circular movements with the ball all around your right inner knee, clockwise and then counterclockwise. This will trigger releases in the tendons of all the muscles that attach at this point.

6. Repeat on the left side.

Routines for the Office, Cars, Planes, and Trains

Whenever you're stuck sitting in one place for hours, you can use these routines to tone your thigh muscles and increase their circulation. When you get up, you won't have tired, stiff legs, but energized muscles that are ready to go!

Use a ball that's small enough to work with comfortably in a chair—about six inches in diameter.

The Hamstrings

This routine brings the ball all the way to the knee joint to compensate for the effects of sitting. Hours of sitting can make the knees stiff, and placing the ball in the knee joint will keep the knee from tightening up.

1. Sitting in a chair, with your back braced against its back, place the ball under your right sitbone and sit like this for 10 seconds.

2. With your left leg bent and the left foot resting flat on the floor, lift your right leg and use your hands to move the ball about a quarter inch toward your knee. Sit with the ball here for 10 seconds. Breathe and sink your weight into the ball.

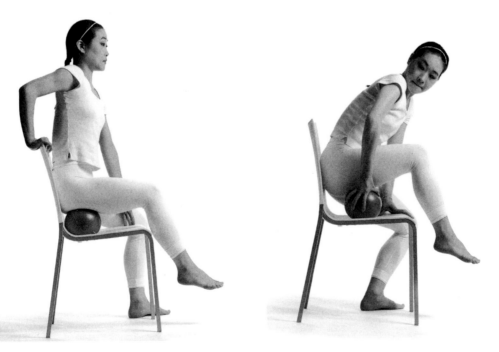

Step 1   Step 2

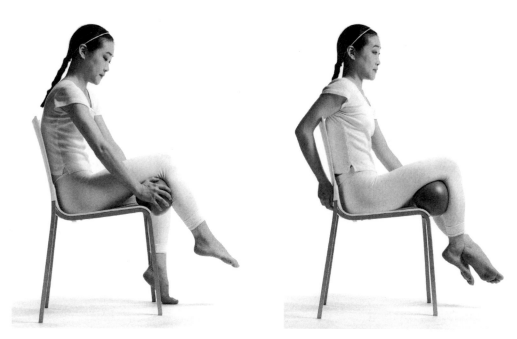

Step 4, ball wedged under knee   **Step 4, left ankle crossed over right**

3. Continue moving the ball forward in quarter-inch increments, keeping it at each point for 10 seconds. When the ball is more or less at mid-thigh (depending on how tall you are), your buttocks will come down to the chair seat. Continue rolling until you reach the knee.

4. Now lift your leg off the chair and with your hands push the ball upward so it's wedged under the knee and pressing against the chair edge. To increase the pressure against the back of the knee, you can cross the left ankle over the right one and use the left leg to pull the right ankle backward (toward you). Keep the ball under the knee for about 30 seconds. This creates space within the knee joint.

5. Repeat on the left side.

Quadriceps

When your knee joint is bent (as it is when you're sitting), you can safely roll all the way to the top of the knee. This way you release the tendons of the quadriceps where they attach to the knee.

1. Sitting in a chair, place the ball in the crease between your right hip and thigh and lean on it with your right elbow or forearm for 10 seconds.

2. Now move the ball about a quarter inch toward your knee. Lean on it again for 10 seconds.

3. Continue to roll the ball down the thigh until you get as close to the knee as you can, pressing into the ball with your elbow or forearm at each point for 10 seconds.

4. Repeat on the left side.

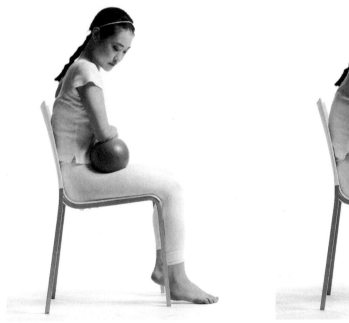

Step 1

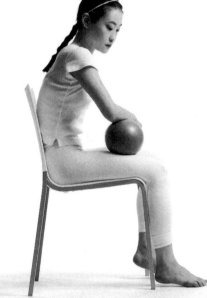

Step 3

Inner Thighs

1. Sitting in a chair, separate your legs so you can place the ball between them, pressing it up against your pubic bone. With your hands, push the ball against the bone. Hold for 5 seconds.

2. Now close your legs, clamping them around the ball. Hold for 5 seconds.

3. Release your legs. With your hands, move the ball a couple of inches toward your knees, then clamp your legs around it again, hold for 5 seconds, then release.

4. Repeat step 3 until the ball reaches your knees.

5. Now place the ball between your knees where they bend at the joint, clamp your knees against it, and hold for 5 seconds.

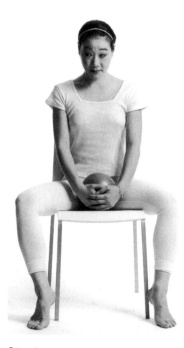

Step 1

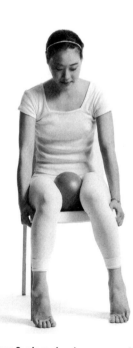

Step 2, clamping legs around ball

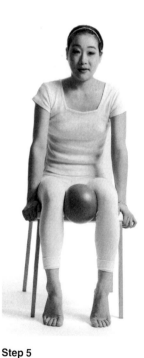

Step 5

7

Feet and Ankles

Your feet are your foundation, like roots into the earth, so your basic interaction with your environment is determined by the way they stand on the ground. As you walk, run to catch a bus, or play sports, all your weight bears down on your feet. When we're young, our feet feel fine; we take them for granted and hardly think about them. Just as with every other part of the body, we're never taught what a healthy foot is and how important it is to keep it healthy. But in fact, well-developed foot muscles and strong arches are essential, for they support the rest of your body and keep you upright—and, of course, shapely well-arched feet are sexy and attractive. What's more, because your feet are quite literally the foundation of every physical action, having strong, healthy feet will enhance everything you do.

Your feet make another important contribution to your appearance. If your feet are weak, you'll never achieve the beautiful body alignment that looks so terrific. No matter how much you work on other parts of yourself, if your feet aren't strong enough to hold you up, they'll collapse. Your ankles will turn in, and the rest of you will go down with them. So be sure to make your feet a part of your workout. Just as you do for the rest of your body, you can strengthen and tone your feet and increase their range of motion. And it doesn't take much: once you get them in good shape, using either of the two simple routines in this chapter, all they need is five minutes once or twice a week.

Quite often I see athletes who appear from the outside to be in perfect condition: strong and with fabulous muscle definition. Yet they've come to me with severe hip pain. When I have them take off their shoes, it turns out they have completely flat feet. The muscles on the bottoms of their feet, whose job is to hold the arches up, are completely undeveloped—and that's the source of the pain. They've worked hard to be perfectly buffed and develop those beautiful arm, chest, and leg muscles. But like many people, they've assumed that their flat feet are inherited, so they've never tried to do anything about them.

It's only when our feet start to hurt—something that can happen at any age, especially because of the shoes we wear—that we realize our feet need attention. The feet are one of the first places in the body where the muscles begin to contract and restrict us as we age, and this affects how the rest of our body moves.

That's why I can't stress enough how important it is to start taking care of your feet while you're young. You won't enjoy your golden years—or any years—if your feet hurt, since you literally won't be able to go anywhere. For most of us, the feet are the most painful part of the body to work on. First, they're the most neglected part; they're confined inside shoes all day, and we hardly ever stretch or massage them as we do the rest of our body. Second, they contain reflex points that affect every other part of our physique. But if you start now and keep at it, in time the foot routine won't be difficult and you'll be able to maintain healthy feet that will give your golden years the chance to live up to their name.

Foot Architecture

The feet support the legs in keeping the rest of the body upright. If your feet are collapsed, your entire body will follow suit in a chain reaction. When your arches are flat, your ankles cave in; your knees collapse inward following the arches; your inner thighs sag downward; your pelvis drops; and your whole spine settles into your lower back and pelvis. People often tell me that they feel their legs are heavy, making it hard to walk, and this is why.

You may be surprised to learn that most of our foot muscles actually go unused. Can you move each of your toes separately from the others? You probably never realized that you have muscles in your feet that should enable each toe to move by itself. Can you fully point and then flex your feet and toes? Many people walk with stiff feet; instead of bending the foot as the toe leaves the ground, they lift each foot and slap it down as a whole. But your feet contain tiny bones that are meant to help them bend naturally as you walk. This flexing of the feet functions as shock absorption. When it's missing, other joints in your body have to absorb that pressure. As a result, those other joints start to wear out.

Most of the foot muscles are at the end of a chain of muscles that begins at the front or back of the knee. If you're not using your foot muscles, you also aren't fully using the related muscles in the calf—which means you're also not fully using the bigger muscles in the thighs. In other words, having stiff feet means that your leg muscles are already in a pattern of contraction. And since even people who work other muscles in their fitness practice routinely forget about the foot muscles, as we've seen, too often they don't fully utilize their feet. Consequently they don't get the most out of their leg workouts, because when the feet aren't working, the leg muscles actually get tighter after a workout, instead of moving more freely.

Foot misalignment is the source of many foot disorders. Bunions, for example, are painful inflammations at the base of the big toe. The base sticks out to the side, while the toe itself angles into the other toes. Women are more likely to get bunions, since they tend to wear shoes with narrow toes or they took ballet lessons as children that got them up on their toes at too early an age. But I believe that bunions are also often caused—in both men and women—by a misalignment that sends all the weight, which should be distributed throughout the foot, into the ball of the big toe. Bunions are usually treated by surgery that cuts away the projecting bone, but since this doesn't change the alignment of the foot, many people still have pain afterward. If people understood the importance of caring for the feet, this wouldn't happen.

SHOES: THE GOOD AND THE BAD

Many people use shoes as a way to take care of their feet. They believe that if you wear the best, ergonomically correct shoes, your feet will be fine. But while it's certainly important to wear rubber soles to cushion your joints from the impact of walking on cement, that doesn't replace caring for your feet in a way that maintains full function in all their muscles and bones.

Sneakers

Huge amounts of money go into designing and manufacturing the best sneakers for different sports. But because sneakers support the foot muscles everywhere, they never get activated and don't do any work. Essentially, when you put on sneakers, you're putting your feet to sleep—then working out. It's great to have these specialized sport shoes, because they're comfortable and they do stabilize the foot and ankle during exercise. But remember that the feet are connected to the rest of the body. If you exercise without consciously working your foot muscles in a way that fully activates the leg muscles they're connected to, you're likely to develop knee and hip problems that ultimately will affect your back. *(continued)*

So make sure your foot bends when you walk, and that you can point and flex your toes, in any pair of sneakers you buy. But beyond that, give your feet their own workout, separately from whatever you do wearing sneakers. That will keep them strong, flexible, and properly aligned.

What About High Heels?

Here's some good news: If your feet are really strong and healthy, you should be able to wear any kind of shoes without permanent damage. It's true that heels—medium as well as high—affect your alignment by shifting weight to the ball of the foot. So you wouldn't want to wear them all day, every day. But you should be able to wear them for short periods without causing foot, leg, or back pain—as long as each time you wear them, you work the negative alignment that heels create out of your whole body, as well as your feet, so you don't get stuck in poor posture patterns.

Thin-Soled Flats

Watch out for flat shoes with thin soles such as loafers, moccasins, and some types of sandals. In these shoes your feet hit the pavement without any cushioning to provide shock absorption. It's best not to make these a daily walking shoe. But if you really like them as a daily shoe, be sure to work on your feet several times a week to restore proper shock absorption and stimulate the muscles that support the arch.

Another common measure for relieving foot problems is an orthotic, a support inserted into a shoe. To me, though, orthotics aren't a cure—they're a Band-Aid. They offer temporary relief, but rather than correcting the structure of the foot, they make the structure dependent on the orthotic. And by keeping the foot in the misaligned position, they actually reinforce the misalignment. Far better to take care of your feet yourself by correcting their structure.

Balls for the Feet

The balls you use for the foot routine are different from the other Body Rolling balls. You need a solid rubber ball (called a sponge ball) about two and a half inches in diameter. It should be firm, not soft. *Don't* use a golf ball or Superball—they're much too hard *and will injure you.* Don't use a tennis ball or any other hollow ball, for it will indent when you put all your weight into it, rather than giving like solid rubber. The best ball I have found is the Pinky, which is widely available at drugstores and chain stores such as Kmart and Wal-Mart. You will need two balls so you can work both feet together.

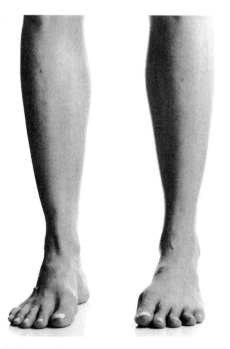

Optimal foot alignment

I've also developed "Foot Savers," plastic half-spheres with flat bottoms that are easier to balance on than balls. Foot Savers allow you to work all the points of the foot in much greater detail. (For mail-order information, see Resources, page 213.)

Optimal Foot Alignment

In the ideally aligned foot

- Weight is distributed equally on the heel, the outside of the foot, and the ball of the foot.

- The arch is lifted.

- The ankles are straight, not collapsed in or leaning out.

- All the toes are fully extended, separated from each other, and relaxed, not gripping the floor to hold you up.

Self-Exam

Most of us tend to stand either with all our weight on the outside of the foot or with more weight pushing into the big toe and inner ankle. In either of these postures, the weight isn't equally distributed over the entire foot. Notice your own tendency as you observe the following points.

- Stand up barefoot. Can you lift all your toes up off the floor together and then, starting with the little toes, place each toe down on the floor separately, without letting the toes touch each other?

- Let all your weight drop into the outside of each foot. Keeping the weight there, roll onto the centers of your heels. Now place the entire ball of the foot and the toes on the floor without letting the arch touch the floor. Can you do this comfortably? If you can, you are distributing your weight equally on each foot.

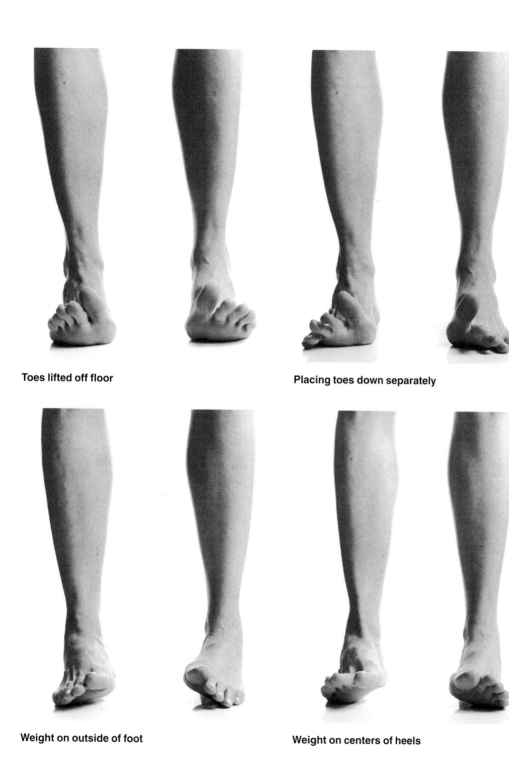

Toes lifted off floor

Placing toes down separately

Weight on outside of foot

Weight on centers of heels

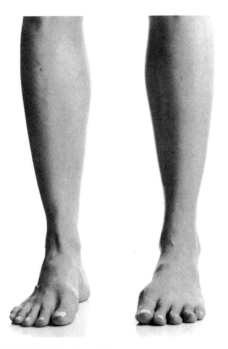

Weight distributed equally

- With your foot in this position of equally distributed weight, can you flatten your toes out on the floor or do the toe knuckles have to bend and grip to keep your foot in this position? Do you feel this effort in other parts of your legs? If so, you are directly experiencing the connection between your feet and the rest of your body and learning how your foot position affects the rest of you.

- Look at your ankles in the mirror. Do they drop inward toward the floor, collapsing your arches? Or are your outer ankles thrust out to the side, putting extra weight on the outside of your foot so that the entire ball of the foot doesn't touch the floor?

Foot Routine

This routine uses two balls, about two and a half inches in diameter, to work the soles of your feet. (You can also use my Foot Savers.) Pressing into the ball sends pressure upward through the leg, reversing any collapse in the feet, stimulating circulation, and reducing swelling in the ankles. A major benefit is that the foot routine will lift and tone your arches, enhancing the shape of your feet. What's more, according to a therapy system called foot reflexology, the sole of the foot contains reflex points that correspond to every part of the body. Stimulating these points helps improve the function of the corresponding organs—so you'll get benefits from this routine throughout your body.

It's best to work both feet at the same time, because that keeps your hips level. If you have trouble balancing on the two balls, stand next to a wall or hold on to a table. Some people's feet are extremely sensitive. If you find it too painful to work both feet together, work one at a time.

This routine is also excellent for arthritis, although you may have to do it sitting down in order to control the amount of weight you put on your feet.

VARIATION 1

This simpler form of the foot routine is good to start out with. These instructions apply to both feet at the same time.

1. Stand with the ball under the center of your heel, with your foot pointing straight in front of you. Hold onto

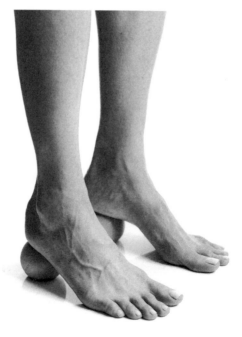

Step 1

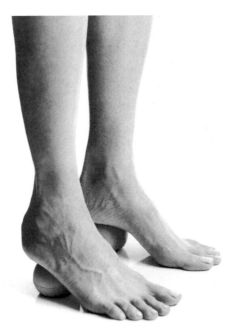

Step 2

the back of a chair, a table, or a wall for balance. Stay like this for 15 to 30 seconds.

2. Microshift your weight, bringing your leg slightly behind you so the ball rolls just off your heel into the beginning of your arch. Part of the ball still touches the heel. You're moving the ball toward your toes, right through the center line of the foot. Let all your weight sink into the ball. Hold for 15 to 30 seconds.

Tips for step 2

- *As you hold, bend your knees a bit to make sure they're not locked. This puts a bit more weight into the ball. But don't let your knees turn in.*

- *It's very important here to keep the arches lifted and the feet pointing straight ahead.*

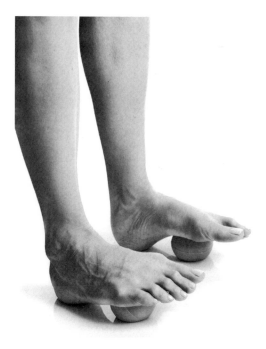

Step 4

3. Now microshift so the ball rolls a bit farther into the arch and hold as in step 2.

4. Continue to roll down the arch, holding at each point, until your weight distribution changes and your heel has to come down to the floor. At this point the ball will be just at the beginning of the ball of the foot, still on the center line.

Tips for step 4

- *The ball of the foot is the padding that makes up the widest part of the foot, just beneath the toes; it extends across the entire foot, from the big toe to the pinky.*

- *Bring one heel down to the floor at a time. This enables you to keep your balance and also to moderate any discomfort. Once the first foot becomes used to standing on the ball this way, bring the other heel down.*

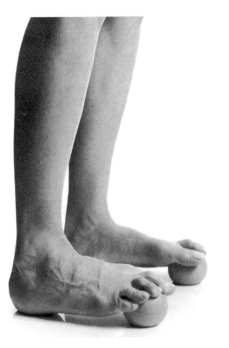

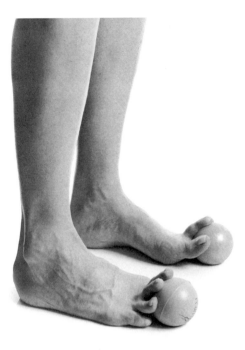

Step 6

Step 7

5. Continue moving the ball forward, working it up over the ball of the foot, toward the toes. Stay at each point for 15 to 30 seconds.

Tips for step 5

- *At each point, move one foot, then the other, to keep your balance.*

- *Remember to bend your knees slightly and consciously sink into the ball at each point.*

6. Continue rolling in small increments until the ball has reached the beginning of your toes and you can spread your toes out over the ball and grip it. Lean your weight into the ball and stay like this for 15 to 30 seconds.

7. Slide the ball out until it reaches the tips of your toes. The ball of the foot is almost on the floor and the toes are stretched out over the ball. Stay here for 15 to 30 seconds.

Tips for step 7

- *Unlike step 6, you're not gripping the ball here; you're letting it stretch out your toes.*

- *If the ball pops out from under your toes, do this step against a piece of furniture or a book braced against a wall.*

8. Now take both balls away and feel for any differences in the way you're standing on the floor.

VARIATION 2

Once you've become used to working the feet with Variation 1, try this variation, which works the sides of the feet separately from the center and will more effectively tone and lift your arches.

1. Follow steps 1 to 5 in Variation 1, except that at each point, after holding for 15 to 30 seconds, move the ball from the center to the outside of the foot. Hold again, then move the ball to the inside edge of the foot and hold. Then bring the ball back to center and roll to the next point. Continue working down the foot this way until both heels are on the floor.

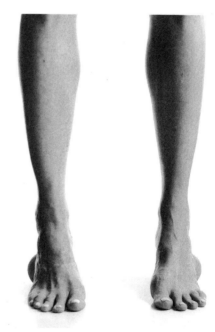

Step 1, ball at outside of foot

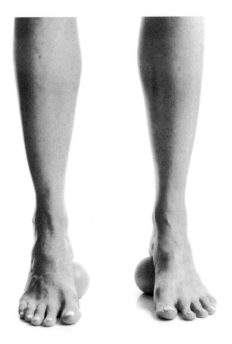

Step 1, ball at inside of foot

Tips for step 1

- *Always move to the outside of the foot first. Working the outside edge raises the arch, making it less painful to press the ball under the inside edge. Also, releasing contraction in the outside foot muscles allows you to stand firmly on that part of the foot and so redistributes your weight, which also helps lift the arch.*

- *Make sure you keep your ankles from turning inward; it's very easy to lose your alignment during this routine. To correct inward-turning ankles, instead of trying to keep your knees straight in front of you, turn them outward. This will keep your ankles from dropping.*

2. When the ball reaches the beginning of the toes, grip it with the three center toes and hold for 15 to 30 seconds (as in step 6 of Variation 1). Then move the ball to the outside edge and

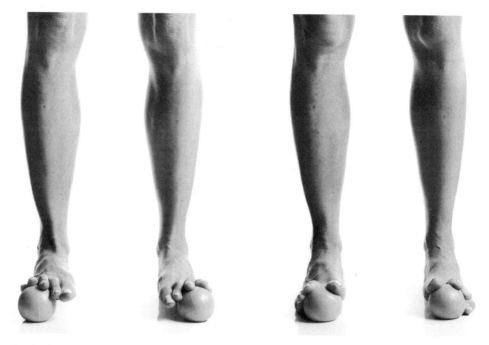

Step 2, gripping ball with last three toes   **Step 2, gripping ball with big toe and second toe**

grip with the last three toes. Finally, move it to the inside edge and grip it with the big toe and second toe.

3. When the ball of the foot comes down to the floor (corresponding to step 7 in Variation 1), stretch the three central toes over the ball, then the outside three toes, and finally the big toe and second toe, holding for 15 to 30 seconds each time.

4. Take the balls away and notice any differences in how you're standing.

8

Neck

We'd all love to preserve the smooth, unlined neck that we have in youth—and the Body Rolling neck routines have exactly this marvelous aesthetic benefit. They'll also give you the long, graceful ballerina neck that's so appealing. And while you're rejuvenating the appearance of your neck, you'll also be working out tight, tense muscles.

How often have you wished that someone was around to rub the back of your neck? The neck is one area where almost everyone feels the buildup of stress. And no wonder—your head weighs about eight pounds, so just carrying it around is a major stress on your neck.

Since the neck vertebrae are the most delicate in the entire spine, this weight subjects them to pressure and compression even before they're affected by poor postural habits and the stress of daily life. That's why neck stiffness is one of the most common body problems we face. Don't we all use the expression, "It's a real pain in the neck"? What's more, tension and shortness in your neck muscles are what will cause lines and sagging skin in this area as you get older.

The skin is essentially the clothing of the muscles, so if your muscles are short and tight, the skin will appear loose and baggy. When your muscles are stretched and toned, your skin will hold its form and not sag and wrinkle (and this is true everywhere in the body). Many women turn to plastic surgery to remove lines and wrinkles from their necks. But you can do the same thing easily, safely, and inexpensively with Body Rolling.

Taking care of your neck is actually quite easy. You need only keep the neck muscles—front, back, and sides—elongated. Rolling your neck out as little as three times a week can prevent a great deal of discomfort and restriction, and you'll reap wonderful aesthetic effects as well.

Firm Up Your Neck

The first sign of contracted neck muscles is lines that develop in the front of your neck. This can occur as early as your twenties. Eventually, these lines will turn into wrinkles. But not to worry—rolling through the muscles in the front of your neck will start to iron out those lines and prevent the wrinkles from forming. By elongating the muscles you can even reverse the effects of aging; you'll have less sagging skin and fewer wrinkles, and any double chin will be diminished. Working all the front-of-neck muscles also keeps the muscles around the mouth and chin more toned—minimizing wrinkles there as well. In this way, Body Rolling makes cosmetic surgery unnecessary.

Often women who have had plastic surgery on their necks come to me for neck stiffness. The surgery pulls back the tissue right behind the jaw, restricting head and neck movement. Women who have this surgery repeatedly reach a point where they can no longer turn their necks easily. What's more, by tightening the front of the neck, the surgery makes the muscles even shorter. So over time, the sagging skin you went to all that trouble and expense to get rid of will return. The way to avoid all this is to strengthen and lengthen your neck muscles to change your head and neck posture.

Common Postures That Cause Neck Problems

Do you recognize yourself in any of these postural portraits?

Head ahead. In the most common misalignment, the head is held slightly in front of the body. Automatically, this position unbalances the neck muscles. The front-of-neck muscles are underused, so they start to atrophy and sag, while the back-of-neck muscles are overused, since they must do most of the work of holding the head up. Because of the strain on these muscles, the trapezius, the heavy muscle that runs along the top of the back, is also overworked and contracts into the hard bulge you instinctively knead when your neck and shoulder hurt.

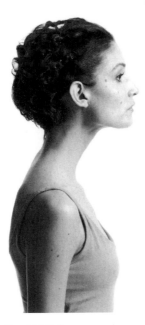

Head ahead

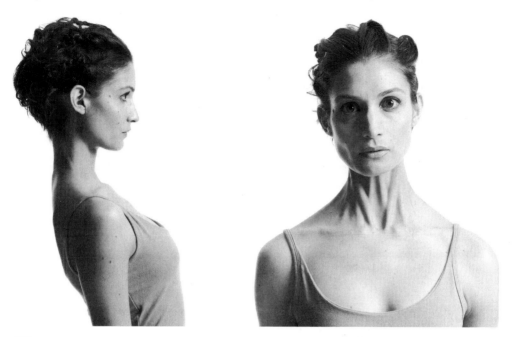

Military pose   **Gripped in front**

The military pose. The opposite position, which chiropractors label the "military pose," is an exaggeration of being upright that actually tilts the torso backward. The back of the neck is completely flat, and the back of the head is held an inch or so behind the rest of the body. This places unnecessary tension on the muscles of the front of the neck and makes the upper body even more stiff.

Gripped in front. The neck is like the shoulders in its ability to collect and hold tension. When people talk, think, or work hard, much of the tension generated by this activity goes into the neck. Think of people who are so intense in a conversation that all the muscles in the front of their neck contract, making the cords stand out. They're completely unaware of how tightly they're squeezing these muscles—and of course they don't realize that this gripping helps limit their neck mobility and underlies any pain they develop in the back of the neck.

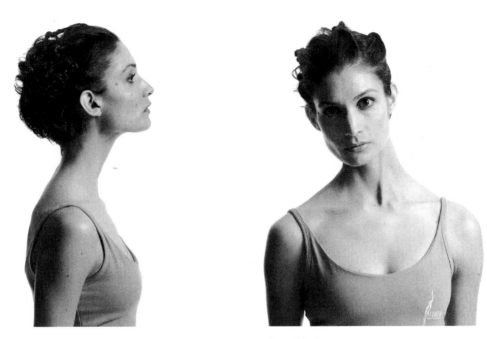

Chin lifted

One-sided

Chin lifted. As women age and develop a double chin, or wrinkles in the front of the neck, they often walk around with their chin lifted to minimize these features. But lifting the chin this way shortens the neck in back, restricting its movement as well as compressing the spine and particularly the disks, which start to protrude and press on nerves—eventually leading to neck, shoulder, and hand pain.

One-sided. People who always hold the phone at the same ear will eventually contract the muscles on that side of their neck, leaving their head permanently tilted to the side. Those whose job requires their neck to be turned or positioned at a certain angle will eventually maintain that position all the time. The upper body will follow, as the muscles on that whole side of the body shorten. People who practice a one-sided sport such as tennis or golf, or who swim the crawl by turning the head only to one side, will shorten their neck in a

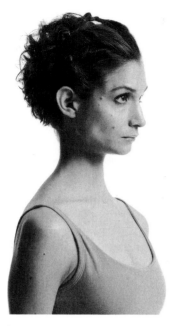

Clenched jaw

similar way. In all these cases, the space between shoulder and head shortens. The difference between that side and the other leads to restricted movement and discomfort.

Clenched jaw. This is an extremely common habit, and no one realizes its harmful effects. Grinding or clenching your teeth is a major contributor to neck tension and restriction. Conversely, if you have temporomandibular joint syndrome (TMJ), or pain in the hinge of the jaw, you can be sure you also have some type of neck problem.

Self-Exam

Ask someone to observe you from the side or use a second mirror to see your reflection as you stand sideways in front of a large mirror.

- Is your neck in line with your shoulders? Or does it protrude in front of your shoulders or press back behind them?

- Where is your chin? Does it tilt up? Point straight out in front of you? Drop down more than just a bit?

- Do you have a double chin? Do you have lots of lines or wrinkles in the front of your neck? Both of these conditions indicate that some of your front neck muscles are not doing their job.

- Can you turn your head to both sides, so that your chin reaches the shoulder on each side? Or does it reach farther on one side than on the other?

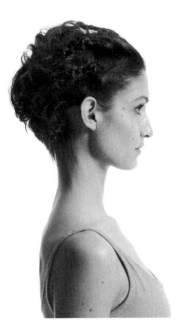

Optimal neck alignment

- Can you comfortably drop your chin to your chest?

- Can you lower each ear an equal distance toward its shoulder, or is there a difference between left and right?

Beginning Your Neck Work

Relieving neck tension and restriction requires working more than just the muscles in the area where you feel discomfort. Since the neck muscles are part of the muscle chain that runs up the back, if the back muscles are tense they will create tension in the neck. So to release the neck, you must start with the basic back routine beginning on page 60. When you place the ball at the base of your spine, you set off a natural release that flows up the spine, so by the time you reach the neck the muscles there are already in a releasing mode. If you just put the ball at the neck instead, you won't get nearly as much relief.

In doing the back routine, simply add the neck routine as part of rolling out each side.

- Be sure to roll all the way up the back of the skull, since muscles that are part of the muscle chain of the back attach up there. Rolling up the back of the skull continues the release of the back-of-neck muscles that you initiated at the sacrum.

- From the top of the skull, roll back down to the middle of the back of the neck.

Now you're ready to begin the neck routines. These routines will relieve tension and tight muscles in the neck, giving it greater mobility. They'll bring your head and neck back to proper alignment and help relieve tension in your shoulders and jaw. Finally, they'll decrease a double chin and minimize wrinkles and sagging neck skin. Throughout these routines, remember to move the ball in small increments and *breathe fully* at each point.

Back of Neck Routine

If you know that your neck holds a lot of tension, start with a small, soft ball (like my green ball) for this routine. Also, people with short necks will find a smaller ball more effective.

1. As you lie on the floor after doing the basic back routine, press the ball against the right side of your neck and let your head fall slightly to the right, putting more pressure on the right side of the spine. Inhale, then sink into the ball as you exhale.

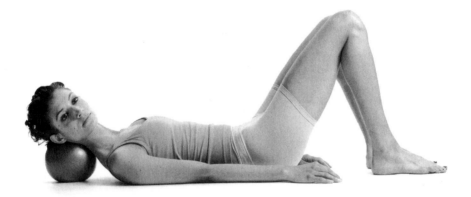

Step 1

2. Inhale and press your head and the right side of your neck against the ball. Your knees are bent and your feet push against the floor to increase the pressure. Maintaining that pressure, use the ball to press into the skin and muscle of the neck. Then, as you exhale, turn your head to the right and continue to press as you slide that skin and muscle toward the ear. Begin to turn your body slowly onto your right side.

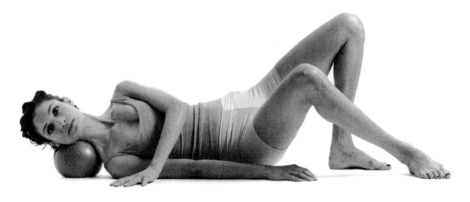

Step 2

3. Continue to inhale and exhale, rolling in micromovements toward the ear. Maintain a firm pressure on the ball and use your left hand on the floor for support while pushing against the floor with your left foot to exert more pressure against the ball.

4. Roll until you are directly on your side, with the ball between the shoulder and the bone behind the ear. Keep your upper right arm directly underneath your body (you can bend your elbow) so that your shoulder remains straight down.

5. Remain on your side for several breaths, relaxing and letting the ball sink into the space between the shoulder and the bone behind the ear.

6. Now, with the heel of your left hand, gently press your head around the ball. At the same time, push the left foot into the

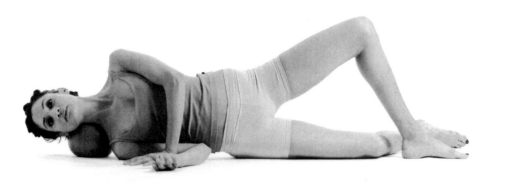

Step 4

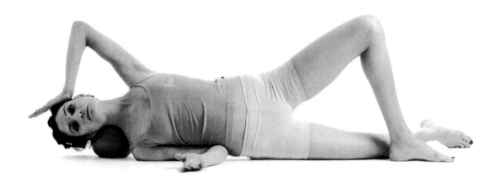

Step 6

floor to scoot your body toward your head. Stay here for a full minute to melt the tension between your head and shoulder.

Tip for step 6

- *This is heaven for the neck: it increases the pressure the ball exerts into the shoulder and neck, stretching and lengthening the side of the neck.*

7. Now slide your right arm and shoulder in front of your body to see how doing so affects the sensation of the ball against the neck.

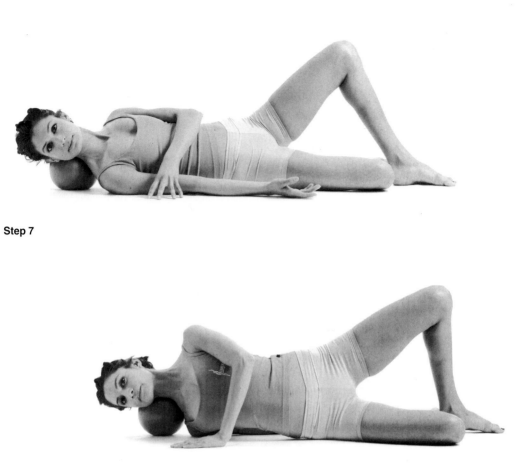

Step 7

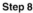

Step 8

8. Next, slide the right arm behind your body and see how that feels. The ball stays in the same position, but the different arm positions release different neck muscles.

9. You can end the routine here, or you can roll back to center, pushing the skin and muscle toward the spine this time. It's very useful and instructive to roll in both directions—sometimes one direction will give much more of a release. In this way you can discover what your neck tension patterns are and figure out how to break them.

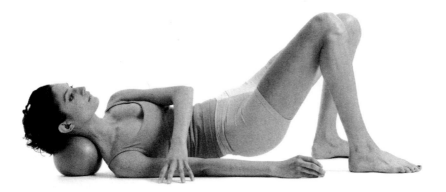

Step 9

Tip for step 9

- *If you like, you can use your right hand to exert pressure on the ball as you roll back to center.*

10. Repeat on the left side of the back and neck.

Front of Neck Routine

This routine begins with a variation of the chest routine in chapter 9 (pages 174–78) to lift the breastbone, which in turn helps lift the front of the neck into correct alignment. You need a relatively soft ball, since it presses directly on bone. Women with large breasts may need a smaller ball (about six inches in diameter), since the ball must fit between the breasts without pressing into breast tissue. Women may need to take their bras off for this routine.

Caution: *Never place the ball at the very bottom tip of the breastbone!* This part of the breastbone is fragile, and putting pressure on it can break it.

1. Lie on the floor facedown. With one finger, feel for the lowest part of your breastbone. Place the ball an inch and a half above the bottom tip of the bone. Let your chest rest over the ball and breathe. Let your head drop toward the floor and use your forearms to support your upper body. Your hips and legs rest on the floor. On the inhalation, feel the back ribs expand; as you exhale, let the ball sink deeper into the breastbone.

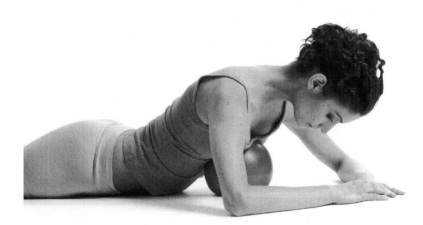

Step 1

2. Scoot your body slightly downward so the ball rolls in a micromovement—about a quarter inch—up the breastbone. Take a full breath as before. Continue to roll up in micromovements. As you approach the top of the breastbone, you'll need to raise your head in order to roll all the way to the top.

3. When the ball reaches the top of the breastbone, hold it so it presses against the two ends of the collarbones.

4. Turn your head as far to the left as you can and lower it so that the ball rests between your jawbone and collarbone. The ball exerts pressure into the entire right side of the neck.

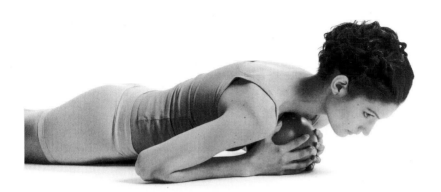

Step 3

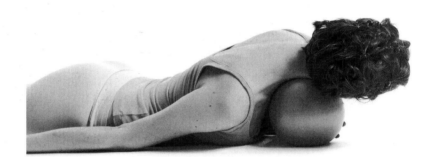

Steps 4 and 5

5. With your left hand, begin to push the ball backward, toward your right ear. Use enough pressure so you feel a stretch in the skin and muscles in the front of your neck. At the same time, move your right shoulder toward your feet and stretch your right arm straight down along the right side of your body. Continue using the ball to push the skin and muscle toward your ear in micromovements.

Tip for step 5

- *For this routine to really work, your left hand must maintain continuous pressure on the ball to intensely stretch the skin and muscle toward the ear.*

6. As the ball approaches the ear, gradually turn onto your right side, bending your knees, until the ball is between your right shoulder and the bone behind your ear, exactly as in step 4 of the previous routine. The right arm is now underneath your body. Stay here, breathing and sinking, pulling your right arm and shoulder away from your neck, for 30 seconds.

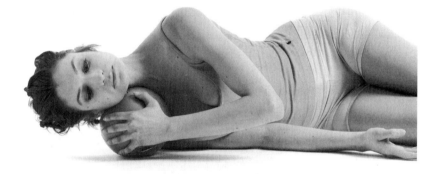

Step 6

7. Now start to roll back toward the center of the front of the neck. Bring your left palm down to the floor at shoulder level for support. Move your right arm behind your body and pull your right shoulder down away from your neck. As you roll slowly back toward the center of the neck, turning to face the floor again, the weight of your head and neck exerts gentle pressure down on the ball so it stretches the skin and muscle along the entire right side of the neck, this time toward your Adam's apple.

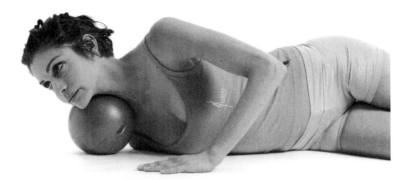

Step 7

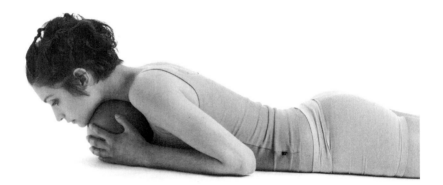

Step 9

Tip for step 7

- *If this is uncomfortable, use your left hand to control the amount of pressure that your head exerts on the ball.*

8. When the ball reaches the center of the neck, (you can roll right up onto your Adam's apple), repeat this routine, starting from step 4, on the left side.

9. When you come back to the center the second time, rest with the ball at the center of your throat. Stay here for 10 to 15 seconds.

- *It may seem scary to let the ball sink right into the center of your throat, but it's safe, and will help release tension in your neck. To control the amount of pressure being exerted on your throat, hold the ball with your hands.*

Concluding Neck Routine

If you're taking the time to work your whole neck, I recommend ending with this routine. It elongates the back of the neck and helps your shoulders drop back and down. It also integrates the back and front neck routines to create maximum length in your spine and your neck muscles.

1. Lie on your back and place the ball right at the center of your neck, at the base of your skull. Your arms lie alongside your body, with your palms facing down, and your shoulders pull away from your head. Bend your legs and press your feet into the floor.

2. Inhale, lifting your hips as high off the floor as you can. Exhale, holding your hips up.

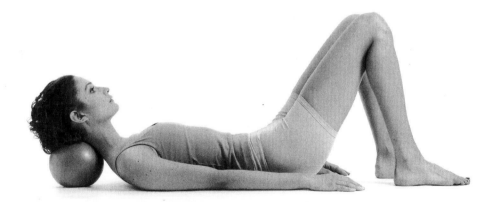

Step 1

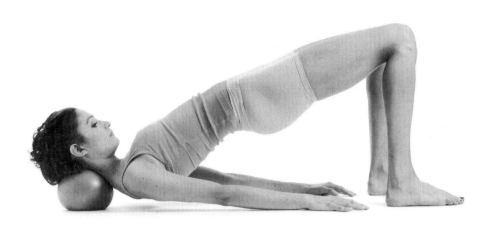

Step 2

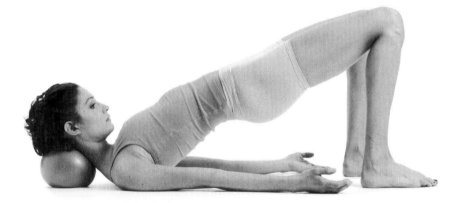

Step 3, working shoulders down to floor

3. Keep your hips lifted as you continue breathing. Lifting your hips will also lift your shoulders off the floor. Now work the shoulders *down* to the floor, *without lowering the hips*, to increase the stretch. At the same time, reach your hands toward your heels; this helps elongate your neck. Meanwhile, push your feet into the floor, pressing your head and neck against the ball. The higher your hips are—with shoulders still touching the floor—the more pressure there is, maximizing the length in the neck muscles.

4. Now lower your hips to the floor and rest for a full breath. Then repeat steps 2 and 3 two or three times. Each time you lift, pull your shoulders a bit farther away from your head and neck.

5. After you lower your hips for the last time, support your head with one hand, take the ball away with the other, lower your head gently, and rest on your back.

9

Shoulders, Arms, and Hands

Have you noticed that the old image of the frail, delicate, waif-like girl isn't sexy anymore? Women are going after a different image today—we want to be strong! We want a beautiful, well-built upper body, with broad shoulders and developed arm muscles—and not a hint of upper-arm flab. When we're strong we feel powerful and attractive, as though we could take on the world. And more than ever, strength is synonymous with beauty. If you don't believe me, just take a look at the latest swimsuit issue of *Sports Illustrated*. Body Rolling will give you this new look—and it will give men the broad chest and shoulders they've desired for years.

What's more, as you use Body Rolling on your shoulders you'll be doing wonders for maintaining a youthful posture. When someone stands up straight, with shoulders squared off and chest open, people immediately see that person as confident, self-assured—and much younger than they really are. Believe it or not, much of our perception of youthfulness derives less from what someone's face looks like than from their posture. Our shoulder position is also related to how we feel about ourselves, for our shoulders are integral to our movements and often mirror our thoughts and emotions. When we're sad or unsure of ourselves, we slouch; when we feel energized and positive, we instinctively throw our shoulders back. For all these reasons, the Body Rolling shoulder routines will bring about big changes in both your physical and emotional well-being.

Where Are Your Shoulders?

Do you know where your shoulders are at any moment? Say you're in a heated argument—intent on taking a firm position, proving your point. What are your shoulders doing? Most likely, they're taking that position, too: hiked up toward your ears and pulled in to your sides. Or you're sitting at your desk at work, thinking out a problem. As you stare at your computer screen and focus your mind, your shoulders round and your head comes forward—without your even realizing it. Our shoulders get involved in almost everything we do. It's not surprising, then, that our shoulders are the part of us that's most susceptible to stress and strain from repetitive patterns of movement.

Almost everyone is likely to raise their shoulders or round them forward to perform certain tasks or in response to particular events. When you're tired, you tend to droop your shoulders forward. Layered on top of these general habits are your own personal patterns of misalignment. Say you always carry a shoulder bag over your right shoulder: that shoulder will be higher than the left one, since its muscles are contracted. When you take that firm position in an argument, you tighten both shoulders, as described above. But your habitually raised right shoulder will go higher than the left one, restricting your ability to turn your neck. Over time, the muscles in the back of your neck will contract, and you may develop neck pain.

For proper shoulder position, the chest should be lifted, so the shoulders can relax. But, as we've seen, the pattern of dropped chest, head jutting forward, and rounded shoulders is the most common misalignment of all. The dropped chest is deeply ingrained in our sedentary culture. Most jobs, for instance, keep us seated and bent forward, and you may find yourself stuck in this position even after you leave the office.

Sports that use the arms differently also create patterns of tension. Golf, tennis, baseball, and other one-sided sports always make one shoulder higher than the other. And everyone—even ambidextrous people—has a dominant side and uses his or her right and left arms differently, which affects the position of the shoulders.

Since the shoulder is a free-swinging joint, every movement of your hand or arm affects shoulder stability. That's why it's important to understand what makes the shoulder joint stable. Since this joint, along with the spine in the back of the neck, controls the entire arm, hand, and fingers, once you achieve correct alignment, optimal muscle function, and full range of motion in your shoulders, your arms and hands will work properly too.

It's easy to correct your shoulder alignment with Body Rolling, and once you do, your posture will improve and your torso, head, and neck will move much more freely. And, when you align your shoulders, you release and activate your arm and shoulder muscles, which not only become toned but automatically achieve that longed-for muscle definition. Once the shoulder muscles are free, any workout you do will work all those muscles in a balanced way, enhancing your performance.

Firm Up Your Arms

The main reason women develop upper-arm flab is that as girls they never learned to use their upper-arm muscles—the biceps and triceps. Even as the new image of the strong woman spreads through our culture, many of us still have the old one embedded in our bodies, since traditionally boys and girls learn to use their shoulders and arms differently. The most common example is the way each throws a ball: boys use their whole shoulder and arm, girls just their forearms and hands. The new focus on girls' sports is changing this pattern, but there is still a strong cultural imprint on girls of the "feminine" way to do things, evident in the most mundane actions. Think of the typical women's motions of knitting, sewing, and crocheting: small movements that don't fully activate the big arm muscles.

But when you roll through your biceps and triceps with Body Rolling, you wake these muscles up and reactivate them, creating well-toned, developed, ballet-dancer arms.

"Pump It Up!"

For men, a broad chest and shoulders have always been sexy. Men go to the gym to bulk up and develop muscle definition. Frequently their workouts create overdeveloped shoulder and arm muscles, and these contracted muscles can lead to tight shoulder joints that are susceptible to injury. Body Rolling elongates the shoulder and arm muscles and aligns the shoulders properly—and this alignment is what enables you to get the broad chest and upper body lift that look so great. What's more, once your shoulders are properly aligned, you'll avoid any future injury.

Optimal Shoulder Alignment

In optimally aligned shoulders

- The muscles of the chest and back are equally balanced in supporting the shoulder joint.

- The arm hangs freely from the joint, its motion unrestricted.

When the chest muscles are well developed and working properly, they hold the front of your body upright, allowing the shoulders to relax back and down. But when you habitually hunch over, these muscles become contracted and short, unable to balance the trapezius, or upper back muscle. With the shoulders curled forward, and the chest muscles not doing their share, the trapezius must work harder and become the major mover of the shoulder. Often it turns into a thick, hard bulge, like a monkey on your shoulder.

When the trapezius and chest muscles are in balance, the arm will also be in optimal position. And when the arm moves freely, the biceps and triceps can work equally. But if the chest muscles are tight and contracted, the arm rotates forward, preventing full range of motion in the shoulder joint. The biceps (the muscle on the front, or palm side, of your upper arm) contracts, and the triceps (the muscle on the back of the upper arm) becomes lax and unable to contract. The resulting overuse of the biceps and underuse of the triceps leads to over- and underuse of the forearm muscles, which in turn affects the hands and fingers. It's this imbalance that over time can lead to repetitive stress syndromes in the hands and wrists. These problems originate in improper shoulder and arm alignment.

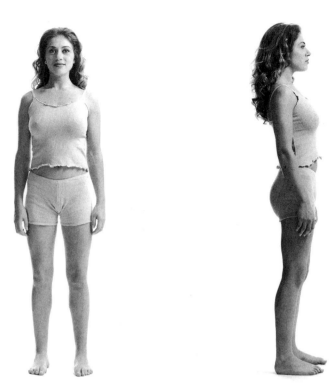

Optimal shoulder alignment, front view   **Optimal shoulder alignment, side view**

Self-Exam

There are many possible types of shoulder misalignment. Here are a few simple points you can observe to discover your personal patterns. Remember that developing an awareness of where your chest and shoulders actually are is the first step to improving your posture.

- The next time you find yourself having an intense conversation on the phone (it's easier to do this when you're not facing another person), pay attention to what your shoulders are doing. Ask yourself: Are my shoulders pulling up toward my ears? Are my arms pulled up into my shoulder joints and pressed against my sides?

- Notice whether you always hold the phone on the same side of your head.

- When you sit down to write or type, ask yourself: What am I doing with my shoulders? What's happening at the place where my arms connect to them? Does my arm pull up into my shoulder and grip to my side? Or does my elbow rotate up and out to the side because my shoulder is pulled forward?

- Notice what happens as you begin to concentrate on a task. Do your shoulders start moving in and up toward your ears? For the next three minutes, stop every thirty seconds and notice whether you're tensing them.

- Do you always carry your briefcase or shoulder bag or your child on the same side?

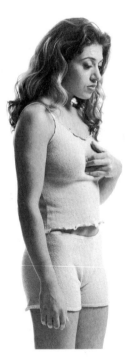

- Where is your chest? To find out, place your fingers an inch below the bottom of your breastbone and gently push downward. What happens to your head and shoulders?

Pushing down on breastbone

- Have someone observe you from the side. Ask that person: Are my shoulders pulled forward or backward? Is my ear right above my shoulder? Do my shoulders hike up, or do they drop down, away from my head and neck? Are my elbows bent, or do my arms drop straight down from my shoulders?

- Can you raise your arms to shoulder level and stretch them straight out in front of you? Out to the sides? Can you rotate your arms through a full circle, straight forward, up overhead, behind you, and back down to your sides? If you answer no to any of these questions, your shoulders are restricting your arm movement.

Exercise: Finding Your Alignment

The following exercise gives you an internal sensation of what proper alignment actually feels like. It provides a specific goal to aim for and also helps you notice more easily when you fall out of alignment.

- Place the fingers of your right hand flat against your chest, just below the collarbone on the left side of your body.

- Slide your fingers out toward the shoulder, while exerting pressure that pushes the shoulder gently backward.

- Now do the same on the other side. You are manually releasing your chest muscles so that the shoulder can move back into its proper alignment.

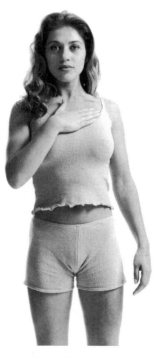

Right hand flat against chest

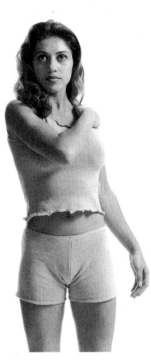

Pressing shoulder backward

If you find you can't push your shoulder back at all, you know that the chest muscles are very tight and really need to be rolled out with the ball.

To realign your shoulder, you should start by lengthening the back muscles with the basic back routine (pages 60–68) in chapter 4. Then do the side and chest routines that follow.

Side Lengthening Routine

You may wonder why we start working on the shoulder with a side routine. I like to say that the shoulder begins in the hip, because in order to properly reposition your shoulders, you need to lift your entire torso. So we work the side of the body to lift the front and back muscles simultaneously. In this way you create the optimal conditions for your shoulder to become properly aligned and then toned. As an added bonus, this exercise is great for getting rid of love handles.

In the side routine, you release the hip joint, then take the ball away, move it up to the rib cage, and roll into the armpit and down the arm to the elbow. Since most people aren't used to working on their side, their rib cage is likely to be quite rigid. The ribs are usually frozen together by the tiny muscles between them, called intercostals, which tend to be tightly contracted. Therefore I recommend that you use a soft ball, nine to ten inches in diameter, or my yellow ball, for this routine.

The side routine will also balance and activate the muscles of the upper arm and forearm. As you roll, keep in mind the image of a tree growing. The muscles of your front and back are like branches that extend outward from a central trunk as they grow upward. The more upright the torso is, the more gracefully and easily they grow. Your goal is to free restrictions in both back and front so that your shoulder and arm can extend outward like these graceful branches. Remember, though, it's your entire torso that's lifting, not your shoulders alone.

> When doing the side routine, *never* roll the ball straight from the hip to the rib cage. In fact, you should never use a ball at all in the space between the hips and ribs.

1. Lie on your right side, with the right leg extended out as long as possible. Hold your torso up with your right palm on the floor. Place the ball under you, at the point where your right leg bone meets your hip joint. Your left knee is bent upward, with the foot flat on the floor, either in front or behind you, for balance. Your left hand is on the floor in front of you.

Tip for step 1

- *If you don't have enough arm or shoulder strength to hold your body up, come down onto your forearm.*

2. From this position, using your hands, slide your body in the direction of your feet, so the ball rolls up in small increments

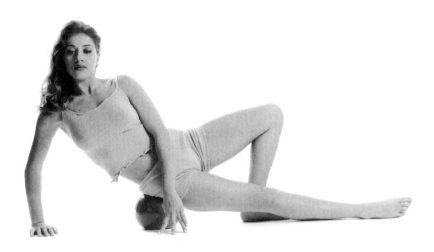

Step 1

to the top of your hipbone. As you roll, breathe and sink into the ball at each point. Continue stretching your right leg out from the hip.

Tip for step 2

- *Keep your torso as upright as you can, so you feel the stretch on your right side. Try to keep your body as much as possible on its side, which means the front of your body doesn't lean forward, and your backside doesn't stick out in back.*

3. Now slowly roll the ball up until it's partly on the hip bone and partly on the muscles just above it. Stay here for a few moments and continue to breathe. As you breathe out, the ball slowly starts to sink into your side just above the hipbone. *It should not be touching the ribs.*

4. With your left hand, pull your ribs up and away from your hips as you breathe. This helps create length between your ribs and hips in the area we often call the "love handles." When the

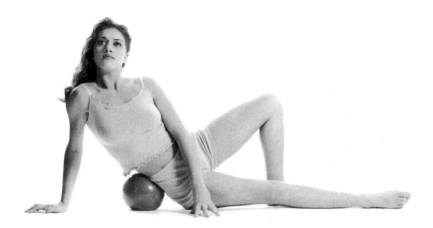

Steps 2 and 3

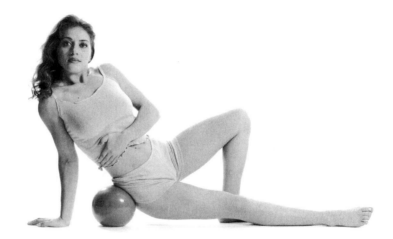

Step 4

muscles here are challenged to stretch, they will gladly oblige, and your love handles will disappear.

5. At this point, sit up. With your fingers, feel for the lowest rib on your right side. Put your little finger on that rib, then place the next three fingers above it. Lie back down over the ball, with the ball placed just above that fourth finger (your index finger).

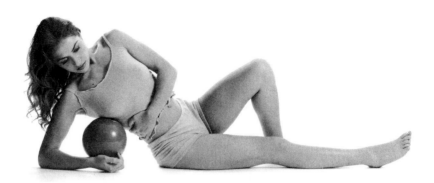

Step 5

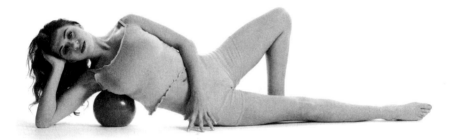

Step 6

Tip for step 5

- *This maneuver is extremely important. It ensures that you are not putting any pressure on your floating rib. The bottom rib on each side is called the floating rib because it's attached to the spine at the back but to nothing at the front, and therefore is extremely vulnerable to being broken.* ***This is why you must never roll straight from the hip to the rib cage.***

6. Continue rolling up the right side of the rib cage, one-half inch at a time, breathing and sinking at each point. Imagine that your rib cage is an accordion expanding and contracting with each breath, opening up the spaces between the ribs.

7. As the ball reaches your armpit, lower your right arm to extend straight out over your head on the floor, and extend your right leg straight out in the opposite direction. Keep your head in a neutral position, looking straight in front of you. If your neck gets tired, cup your left hand over your right shoulder as a pillow to rest your head on. In most people the upper two or three ribs are extremely tight and rigid and will restrict shoulder mobility, so stay at this point for two or three breaths, releasing this area as much as you can.

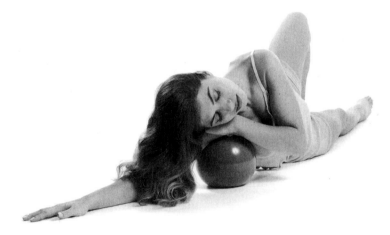

Step 7

8. Now roll the ball farther into the armpit, making sure it's right in the center, not toward the front or back. Your goal is to work toward getting the palm of your extended right arm flat on the floor, stretching the fingertips away from the body. Continue to breathe and sink.

9. Roll the ball a bit higher into your armpit, toward your arm. This is the point where all the muscles of the shoulder girdle

attach to bone, and for many people it's an area of tremendous tension. If you can, stay here and breathe for two or three full breaths.

Tip for step 9

- *You may feel a sensation of pins and needles in your arm, down to your fingertips. This means that your shoulder is extremely tight. Don't worry—the sensation will stop when you release the pressure.*

10. Roll the ball out along your arm, still keeping your palm down on the floor as much as possible. Your whole right side is extended, with the leg and arm still stretching away from each other. The ball is between the biceps and triceps, stretching both of these muscles. As you breathe, feel this entire side elongating.

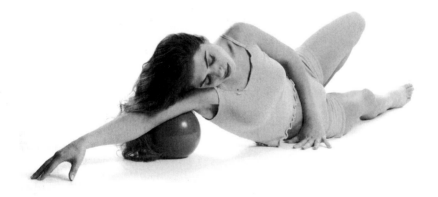

Steps 10 and 11

11. Roll farther down the right arm toward the elbow, breathing and sinking as you go. As you approach the elbow, your right hand and arm will come up off the floor slightly.

12. Now rotate the right hand counterclockwise until the palm faces up. You are now putting pressure into the biceps. Lean

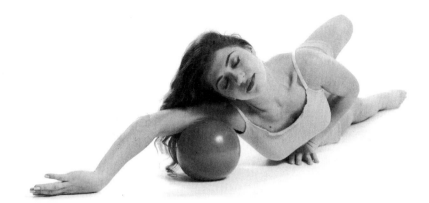

Step 12

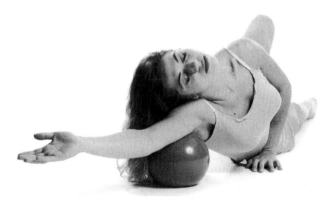

Step 13

your head and chest slightly over your left hand to come more directly onto the biceps. Breathe and sink for another breath.

13. When the ball is halfway to the elbow, rotate your hand clockwise so the palm faces up again. This allows the ball to roll into the triceps. Stay here and breathe for one full breath, putting direct pressure into the triceps.

14. With your palm still facing up, roll the ball onto your elbow bone. Now you can take the ball away and sit up.

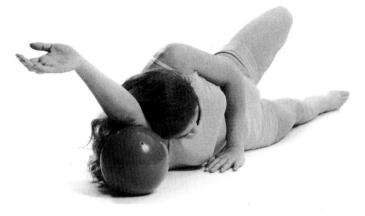

Step 14

15. Stand up and close your eyes. Feel the difference between this side of your body and your left side. Walk around a bit and see if you can feel a difference in the way the two sides move.

16. Look in the mirror and notice any visual differences between the sides. Is the right side of your rib cage breathing more fully? Can you observe a difference between your two shoulders? Has the space between your rib cage and hips changed on the right side?

17. Repeat on the left side.

Chest Routine

I've developed two versions of the chest routine, which works the two major chest muscles (the pectoralis major and minor), elongating and strengthening them to give you perfect upper-body posture—that lifted, self-confident, strong, and sexy stance. After you do this routine for a while, you'll find you just can't slouch anymore.

The first version, which you do on the floor at home, is more effective, because it puts all your body weight on the ball. The second version can be done standing up against the wall in your office. I can't emphasize enough the importance of taking two minutes from every hour to do it, if at all possible. You'll be amazed by the decrease in stress and tension in your neck and shoulders. My clients who follow this practice tell me it's changed their lives: they're more alert and energetic, their posture improves, and they have less lower back pain.

For both these routines, you should use a soft six-inch ball.

CHEST ROUTINE ON THE FLOOR

1. Lie facedown. With one finger, feel for the lowest part of your breastbone. Place the ball an inch and a half above that spot. Let your breastbone press into the ball as you take some of your body weight on your forearms, hips, and legs. Your head should be dropped forward and relaxed. Really concentrate on your breathing. As you inhale, feel your back ribs expand; as you exhale, feel yourself sink into the ball.

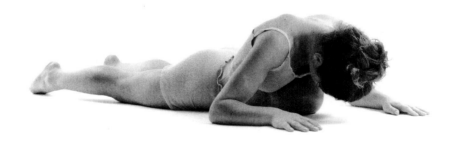

Step 1

Tip for step 1
- ***Do not place the ball at the very bottom tip of the breastbone.*** *This part of the breastbone is fragile, and putting pressure on it can break it.*

2. Move the ball up your breastbone in small increments, about one-quarter inch at a time, breathing and sinking at each point, letting your weight bear down into the ball. Continue until you reach the upper third of your chest. (Women should separate their breasts so the ball does not press on breast tissue.)

3. When the ball is just below your collarbone (women: make sure it is also above breast tissue), extend your right arm out at shoulder level, while twisting your head to the left. Use your left hand to support you on the floor at shoulder level. Inhale, exhale, and sink into the ball.

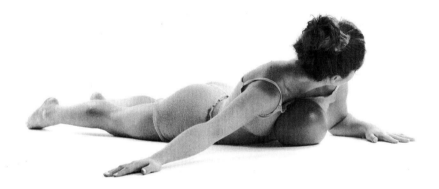

Step 3

4. As you exhale and sink, microshift the ball out very slightly to the right, rolling along the underside of the collarbone. Continue breathing, and each time you exhale and sink, slide the ball slightly to the right, toward the shoulder.

5. When the ball reaches the end of your collarbone, brace yourself on your left hand and begin turning your torso to the left, while raising the torso slightly. With each exhale, sink and twist a bit more to the left, until the ball has rolled right to the point where the right shoulder turns into the arm.

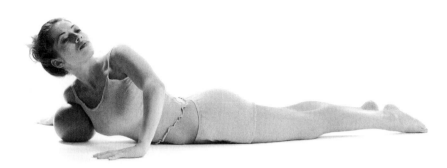

Step 5

6. Now roll the ball down into your arm, twisting your torso more to the left and raising it slightly more at each point, as you look up and to the left. Roll along the biceps, about two-thirds of the way to the elbow.

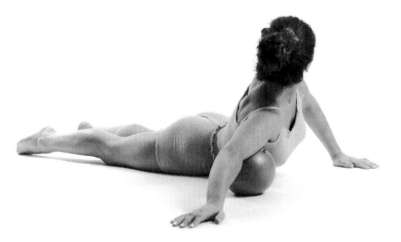

Step 6

7. After rolling the right side, look in the mirror and see if you can observe any differences between the right and left sides of your neck and shoulders. Is the right side of your chest broader?

Is the right shoulder dropped back and down? Is the right side of your neck longer? Notice any difference in your breathing between the right and left sides of your chest.

8. Repeat the routine on the left side.

CHEST ROUTINE AGAINST THE WALL

Take your shoes off (unless you're wearing rubber soles) and make sure your feet won't slip on whatever surface you're standing on; you may need to take your socks off as well.

1. Face the wall and stand with your feet about a foot and a half to two feet from the baseboard (depending on your height). Place the ball against the upper part of your breastbone, just below your collarbone. Women should make sure the ball is above breast tissue.

2. Extend your right arm out against the wall at shoulder level, and twist your head to the left. Put your left hand on the wall for support. Inhale, and as you exhale sink your body weight into the ball by leaning into it.

3. Take a small step to the left and roll the ball out toward your right shoulder in a micromovement, as you continue to twist your head and torso toward the left. Maintaining the twist against the pressure of the ball stretches the chest muscles and pushes the shoulder back.

4. Continue to breathe and, with each breath, microshift the ball farther toward your right shoulder.

5. When the ball is at your shoulder, shift your weight so that your entire torso turns toward the left and both feet are facing left. This puts more direct pressure into the shoulder joint.

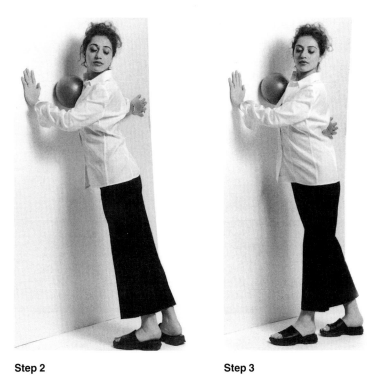

Step 2

Step 3

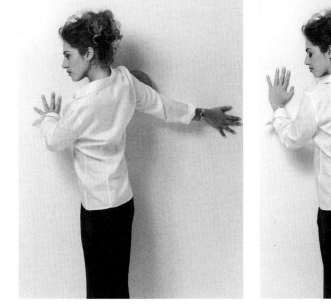

Step 5

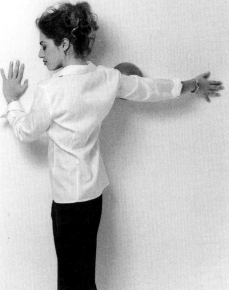

Step 6

Your right arm is extended at shoulder level along the wall behind you.

6. Continuing to inhale, exhale, and sink, roll the ball bit by bit along your right arm, rolling along the biceps. You're now facing completely left, stepping your right foot forward in line with the left foot.

Tip for step 6

- *Make sure you keep your arm* at shoulder level *as the ball rolls along the arm.*

7. Continue until the ball is about two-thirds of the way to the elbow.

8. Repeat on the left side.

Gentle Shoulder Release

This is a really soothing, relaxing way for anyone to open his or her shoulders.

1. Lie on a bed on your right side, with your right arm hanging off the bed and the ball wedged between the edge of the bed and your armpit.

Tip for step 1

- *Make sure the ball is really in your armpit, not pressing into your upper ribs.*

2. Reach your left arm across and cup your left hand around your right shoulder. Rest your head on the back of your left hand. This supports the neck.

3. Stay in this position for 30 to 60 seconds, moving the ball slightly to the front and then the back of the armpit.

4. Repeat on the left side.

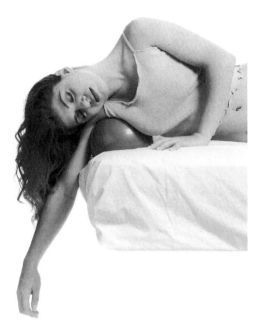

Step 1

Frozen Shoulder Routine

If you can't raise your arm sideways to shoulder level without your whole shoulder lifting, chances are you're starting to develop a frozen shoulder. In this condition the muscles and bones of the shoulder joint freeze together, preventing full arm movement. This routine will help unfreeze the joint. An eight- to ten-inch ball is best because it creates more space in the joint. If you have pain in your shoulder, however, start with a smaller ball, then graduate to a larger one.

1. Raise your right arm out to the side and use your left hand to push the ball up into your armpit as firmly as you can. Relax your right arm down over the ball. Reach in front of your body with your left hand, grab your right wrist or forearm, and pull it to the left. This action locks the ball into your armpit. Pull

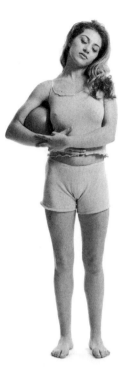

Step 1

your right shoulder down away from your head and neck and stretch your left ear toward your left shoulder.

Tip for step 1

- *Your right elbow should not rotate in front of your body but should remain directly out to the side.*

2. As you inhale, your ribs will expand out against the ball; as you exhale and the ribs move inward, pull your right arm more strongly against the ball with your left hand.

3. Even if you are only experiencing stiffness on one side, be sure to do this routine on both sides for balance.

10

Body Rolling for Older People

In a large Body Rolling class in California, I was teaching people of many different ages to work the front of the torso. Just as in chapter 9 of this book, I explained that this routine would help lift the breastbone and open the shoulders, reversing the aging posture. People spend so much money on facelifts, rejuvenating drugs, and other ways to be more youthful, I said, but they don't do anything about their posture, which is so basic and can change your entire way of being in your body.

When the class was over, an excited woman came up to me. She was about seventy, and had obviously had a facelift. "Look at how I'm standing!" she exclaimed. "I'm not standing like an old person! When you were talking about that aging posture, something just snapped me open. I've spent so much time and energy trying to be young. And now suddenly I feel like I am young—my shoulders are back, my chest is up and open, my head isn't forward!"

Somehow, it had come through to her loud and clear that her attention had been on the wrong things, and that she could break out of her habitual downward slouch. And when she did, she discovered a whole new freedom and ease in her body that she hadn't dreamed was possible despite all her efforts to *look* young.

As this woman learned, Body Rolling means that you don't have to get stiff as you grow older. Most people begin living with daily discomfort and restrictions as they pass sixty; a primary example is the neck. You've seen people who turn the whole upper part of their body around because they can't turn their head by itself. The classic situation is not being able to look back when you're driving, but being unable to turn your head makes many other actions difficult as well.

People tend to accept these changes as inevitable, particularly because they represent a problem for which medicine is unlikely to provide much relief. The average doctor's attitude will often be, "So you can't turn your neck all the way around—that's no big deal, you're getting older." You simply learn to live with your limitations, as long as you can get by every day. But in fact, there are certain simple capabilities that you shouldn't ever have to lose—like turning your neck all the way to both sides, or raising your arm over your head. Turning your neck should be something you can do for your whole life.

And with Body Rolling, you can. It will keep you active, prevent stiffening, even bring back mobility you may have lost. Your muscles and bones stay supple and toned, so that your body doesn't hold you back from living your life. Many people can't wait to retire so they can enjoy themselves after working hard for many years. But when I talk to retired people, they often say, "This isn't so great. My feet, my neck, my shoulder hurt me." The biggest thing keeping them from doing all the things they dreamed of with their free time is their body.

Older people who are less active and mobile can also benefit from Body Rolling. In fact, it's great for anyone—no matter how old they are or what their physical condition is. The most fundamental effect of the routines is to increase circulation and mobility—something everyone needs. And because Body Rolling is a passive form of work-out that uses your own body weight as resistance, it's ideal for people who can't be very physically active.

This chapter offers a range of modified ways to do the routines, depending on your level of mobility and flexibility. There are modifications for healthy, active people over seventy and others for those confined to a bed or chair. The bed and chair routines are also great for people of any age depending on their physical abilities. If you can't stand up to do the foot routine, for example, you can do it in a chair (see pages 204–208). These routines are also excellent for people who are paralyzed, recovering from a stroke, or in bed recuperating from surgery.

After getting comfortable with the basic back and hamstring routines, an older person might want to focus on a particular area where gaining flexibility would make a big difference. For example, after my older clients work on their neck for a while, they're often amazed to find that they can turn their head farther in both directions than they have been able to do for ten years. This unanticipated freedom gives them a whole new lease on life.

Be aware that if you've had your misalignment patterns for a long time, you may not be able to change them completely. But if you use Body Rolling to keep the affected muscles from contracting further, you can prevent these patterns from getting completely hardened and avoid much discomfort or even disability.

Caution: *Since the front and sides of the rib cage are the parts of the body that break most easily, older people should not begin by doing Body Rolling in these areas. Instead, these should be the last areas that they work with. Be sure to do any routine in which the ball touches these parts of the rib cage with great caution.*

Basic Back and Hamstring Routines

The parts of the body that you require for basic mobility are the spine and the legs, so that's where an active older person can begin Body Rolling. Anyone who can get down on the floor can safely do the basic back routine and the hamstring release. These routines don't require much arm strength to hold you up.

Many people can work on the ball quite well once they're on the floor, but getting there can be a challenge; some are also afraid that once they're down they won't be able to get back up. If this is a problem, make sure you're near a doorknob, a table leg, or a low table or chair that you can hold on to as you lower and raise yourself. People who have difficulty balancing or holding themselves upright on the ball can use a wall for support; you'll find a separate section in the instructions that follow that explains how to do this.

Always use a soft ball for the routines in this chapter, and follow the instructions for pacing your breathing given in chapter 3 (page 53).

The Basic Back Routine

Since keeping the spine healthy and flexible is the key to slowing down the aging process, the basic back routine is a necessity for older people. The routine starts with a simple release of the hamstrings (the muscles at the backs of the thighs) before you actually start rolling up the back.

1. Place the ball under the right sitbone (for instructions on finding your sitbone, see page 49), with the right leg extended straight out. Bend the left knee up, keeping the left foot flat on the floor to help you to balance on the ball and to move. Use your hands or fingertips on the floor to help support you and for balance. Roll the ball forward and backward, then side to

side on the sitbone. Roll clockwise, then counterclockwise. Your right leg will bend a bit as you move the ball around the sitbone.

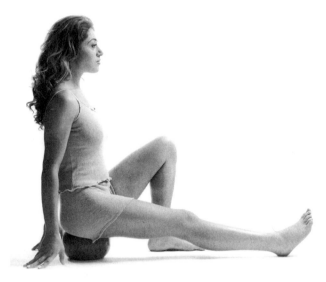

Step 1

2. Using your fingertips and left foot, pull your body behind you and roll the ball a couple of inches down the back of your leg. Take a full breath in and let the back of your leg sink into the ball as you exhale, elongating the hamstrings. Roll the ball a couple of inches down the leg two or three more times, breathing and sinking each time. Stop when you're about two-thirds of the way to the knee. Then roll the ball back up to the sitbone in one smooth movement.

Tip for step 2

- *Your fingertips move either in front of you or behind you to help you move the ball down your leg. The tighter your hamstrings are, the farther behind your torso your fingertips will be. If your hamstrings are more flexible, your fingertips might be beside your hips or even in front of them.*

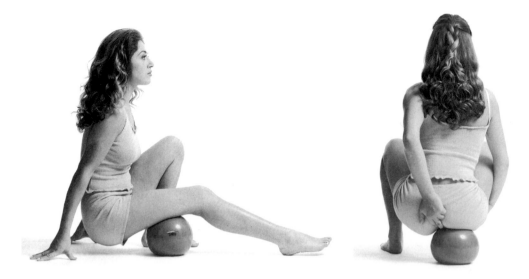

Step 2

Step 3

3. Now you're ready to begin rolling up the back. With the fingers of your left hand, feel for the tailbone—the last bony piece of the spine that you can feel. Roll the ball from the right sit-bone up to the right side of the tailbone. Your knees are bent, both feet are flat on the floor, and your fingertips are on the floor behind you.

    *Caution: Roll to the right side of your tailbone, then up that side. **Never** put your weight on the bottom tip of the tailbone.*

4. Move your body slightly forward and roll the ball a quarter inch up the right side of the sacrum, the flat, pear-shaped bone at the bottom of the spinal column. The ball should be pressing into bone, not muscle. Now, really concentrate on your breathing: inhale, and as you exhale sink your weight into the bone.

5. Continue to roll in micromovements up the right side of the sacrum. You are trying to stimulate the bone itself.

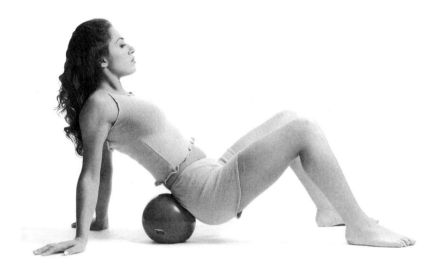

Step 5

Tip for step 5

- *To get the most out of the back routine as a whole, take as much time as you can working your sacrum, sinking as deeply as you can into the ball. The sacrum is where the small muscles of your back begin, and stimulating these tiny muscles at this point sets off a release up the entire back. This stimulation will also improve bone quality and wake up the nerve roots.*

6. When the ball reaches the top of your sacrum, slowly roll it up off the sacrum and onto the right side of the bottom vertebra of your lower back. Inhale deeply, then exhale slowly, sinking your weight into the ball. Now, in micromovements, start to roll the ball slowly up the right side of your spine, taking a full breath at each movement as described in chapter 3 (page 53). Your feet push against the floor to help you move, while your hands help you balance. Your intention is to lift each vertebra away from the one below it and to stimulate and elongate the small muscles.

Remember: The ball should be pressing into the right side of the vertebrae all the way up the spine in order to release the tiny spinal muscles. *Don't roll* across *the spine.*

Tips for step 6

- *You know you're at the top of the sacrum when you feel that you're at the top of your pelvic bone.*

- *Each deep inhalation lifts you slightly off the ball. Each exhalation deflates you so your body sinks heavily into the ball. You'll know when your muscles let go because on the exhalation, the body will sink deeper into the ball. At tight spots, you might want to stay for several breaths.*

7. As you roll slowly up the lower part of the right side of your spine, start to curve your buttocks down and around the ball. Meanwhile, as you inhale, feel your back expand out to where the ball is; as you exhale, sink down into the ball. Your buttocks are gradually dropping toward the floor.

8. When your buttocks reach the floor, the ball will be fully supporting the entire lower spine. Now raise your hands to gently support your head so it doesn't drop backward. If you feel you're losing your balance, use one hand to push the ball into your lower back as the other hand supports your head and neck.

Tip for step 8

- *At no time should your head drop back unsupported. Use one hand to support your head, leaving the other hand free to keep you balanced.*

9. Sliding forward, continue to roll up the right side of your back, one inch at a time. At each point, exaggerate your inhale so you feel your back pressing out into the ball. At each exhale sink into the ball. At the *end* of each exhalation, slide the ball up the

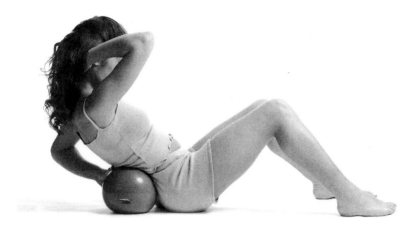

Step 8

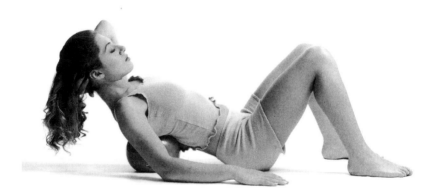

Step 9

next inch. Continue until the ball is at shoulder level, pressing against the right side of the spine, between the spine and the shoulder blade.

Tip for step 9

- *As you roll, your abdominal muscles may begin to quiver, indicating that they need strengthening. As you continue doing this routine, they will indeed grow stronger, since Body Rolling offers powerful abdominal strengthening and core balance.*

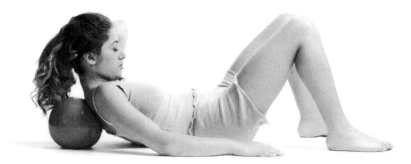

Step 10, chin to chest

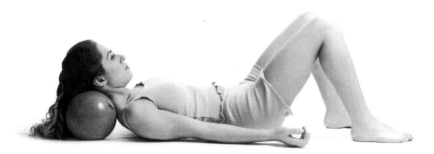

Step 10, head and neck resting around ball

10. Now pull your head all the way forward with your left hand. Bring your chin to your chest and roll the ball up into the right side of your neck. Let your neck and head come to rest against the ball. Your chin should remain pointed down toward your chest. Try to lower your right shoulder to the floor and pull it toward your feet. Your right palm faces the ceiling.

Tip for step 10

• *Pulling your chin toward your chest keeps the back of the neck elongated and straight on the ball. Don't turn your neck—turning prevents you from fully elongating your neck muscles.*

11. Continue inhaling and exhaling. As you inhale, feel the right side of your neck pressing out into the ball; as you exhale, feel it sinking into the ball. Now return to micromovements, trying to move the ball in tiny increments up the back of your neck. Be sure to keep your head straight; don't turn it off to one side.

Tip for step 11

- *If you can't keep your head straight, it's because your neck muscles are tight. As you continue doing this routine, those muscles will release.*

12. When the ball is just below the right side of your skull, feel it pushing up against the bony ridge at the bottom of your skull. Imagine that you're separating your skull from your neck. Keep scooting forward; as you do the ball will roll up onto the right side of the back of the skull. Roll up to the very top of the back of your head, continuing to pull your right shoulder away from your head. Use your left hand to hold the ball so it doesn't pop out from under you.

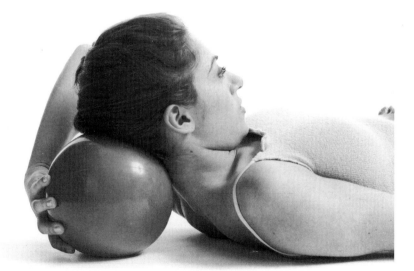

Step 12

13. To finish, support your neck with your right hand, roll the ball out from under you with your left hand, and use your right hand to slowly lower your head. Extend your legs out on the floor, arms alongside your body. Take a couple of deep breaths and notice any difference you feel between this side of your body and the left side.

14. If you have time, stand up and walk around, noticing the difference between the sides as you move.

15. Repeat the routine on the left side.

Hamstring Release

This version of the hamstring release is more detailed than the one that begins the basic back routine. There are three hamstring muscles; two attach at the inner knee, and the third attaches at the outer knee. Step 6 works the whole muscle group; steps 7 and 8 work the outer hamstring; and steps 9 and 10 work the two inner ones. This routine will show you which of your hamstring muscles is tightest.

As you roll down the hamstrings, you should feel the weight of your body pressing down into the ball, which at the same time exerts pressure up into the leg muscles. This routine actually irons out the hamstring muscles, which you will experience as a sensation that the muscles are stretching out. You might not feel the full effect of rolling down your leg until you get off the ball, stand up, and walk around. It's then that you will really see and feel the changes.

1. Place the ball under your right sitbone, sinking all your weight into it. Use your hands or fingertips on the floor to help support you and for balance. Your right leg extends straight out in front of you; the left leg is bent, with your left foot flat on the floor. The left leg helps you balance and move on the ball. Your right leg will bend a bit as you move the ball around the sitbone.

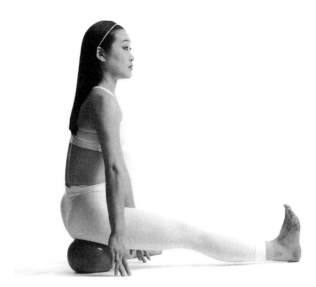

Step 1

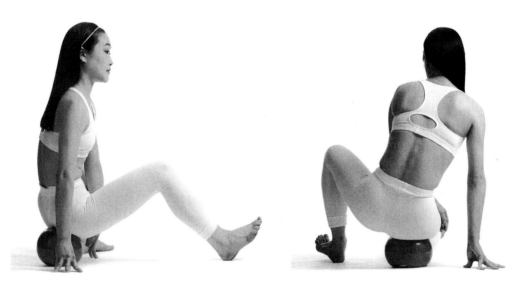

Step 2, rolling forward

Step 3

2. Gently move your body forward and backward so the ball rolls behind, then in front of, the right sitbone. Use your fingertips and left foot to shift yourself forward and backward.

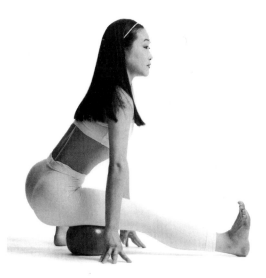

Steps 5 and 6

3. Now shift your body weight from side to side on the ball, building up momentum so the ball rolls from one end of the right sitbone to the other end.

4. Roll clockwise and counterclockwise around the right sitbone.

5. Now, using your fingertips and left foot, pull your body backward and roll the ball a couple of inches down the back of your right leg. Take a full breath in and as you exhale, let the back of the leg sink into the ball, stretching the hamstrings.

6. Continue to roll the ball forward in two-inch increments, sinking and waiting at each point, about two-thirds of the way to your knee. Then roll the ball back up over the hamstring muscles to the sitbone in one smooth movement.

Tip for step 6

- *If you can't roll the ball back up over your hamstrings, use your hands to take it out from under your leg and place it back under your sitbone.*

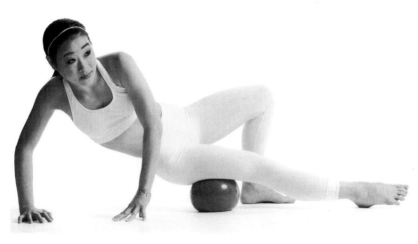

Step 8

7. Now roll the ball forward off the sitbone and shift your weight to the left, so the ball rolls to the right side of the back of your right leg just below the sitbone. Place both your hands on the floor on your right side. Lean on your hands for support as you turn the leg out to the right.

8. Pull your body backward and roll the ball a couple of inches down the leg, leaning to the right side so you're putting more weight into the outer hamstring muscle. The ball is rolling down the outside of the back of your thigh. Continue rolling in two-inch increments, to about two-thirds of the way to the knee.

Tip for step 8

- *Don't turn all the way onto your side here; if you do, you won't be on the hamstring anymore.*

9. Roll the ball back up to the right sitbone as you straighten up-ward. Now keep the weight of your body between your legs

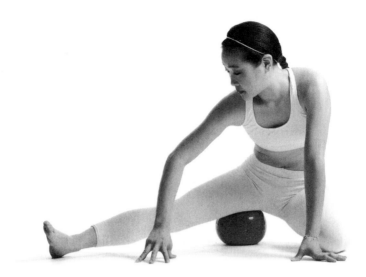

Steps 9 and 10

and place your hands on the floor in front of you, between your legs.

If you have difficulty turning your leg in and out in steps 7 to 10, just stick with steps 1 to 6 for a while, until your hamstrings loosen up and you become more flexible.

10. Roll the ball off the sitbone, turn your right leg inward, and slide the ball slightly to the left, to the inside of the back of your thigh. The ball is now on your inner hamstring. Keep your leg turned inward as you bring your left knee down to the floor and turn it out slightly to the left. Then roll toward the right knee in two-inch increments as before.

Tip for step 10

- *If it's difficult to feel the two inner hamstring muscles, turn your left knee out a little farther to the left. You can also try leaning your torso more to the left as you bend forward.*

11. Repeat the entire routine on the left side.

Seated Wall Variations

If you have difficulty sitting and balancing on the ball, these variations use the wall to keep you from wobbling. One is for the hamstring release, the other for the beginning of the basic back routine.

Hamstring Release Against the Wall

1. Sit with your back leaning against the wall and the ball under your right sitbone. Extend your right leg in front of you and bend your left leg, with the left foot flat on the floor to support you.

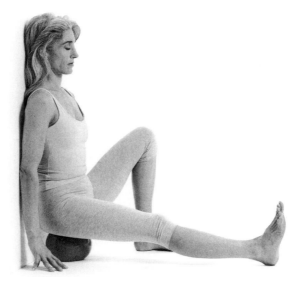

Step 1

2. Push down with your left foot, and shift your weight to the left, still leaning your back against the wall. As you do this your right sitbone lifts off the ball just enough to allow you to slide the ball down your thigh with your right hand. Move the ball in two-inch increments toward your knee. Your buttocks will

drop toward the floor as you approach the knee, but the wall will keep your back straight.

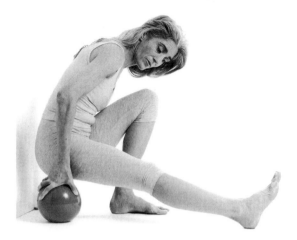

Step 2

3. Once your buttocks are on the floor, it's easy to continue moving the ball down your thigh as in the regular routine.

4. Repeat on the left side.

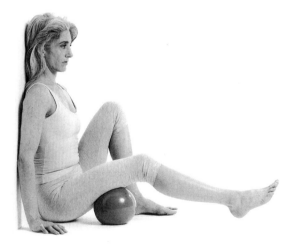

Step 3

Back Routine Against the Wall

If you can't sit balanced on the ball, can't put weight onto your hands or wrists, or your abdominal muscles are too weak to hold you up, this is a great way to get the benefits of the back routine, with a little support from a wall. You should use the same slow, rhythmic breathing and sinking as in the regular back routine.

1. Sit with the ball under your right sitbone and your back against the wall. Your legs are bent, with your feet flat on the floor.

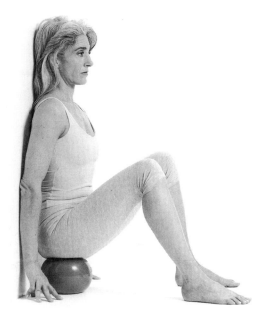

Step 1

2. Leaning against the wall, slide forward to roll the ball up to the bottom of your tailbone on the right side.

   Caution: **Never roll the ball onto the tip of the tail- bone—the pressure can cause the bone to break.**

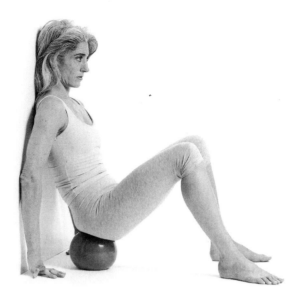

Step 2

3. Continuing to slide forward, begin to roll the ball up the right side of your sacrum, keeping your back against the wall. Your feet help push your body into the ball and keep you balanced. You will need to walk your feet forward as you go.

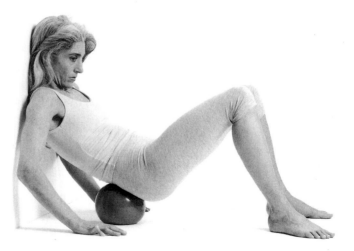

Step 3

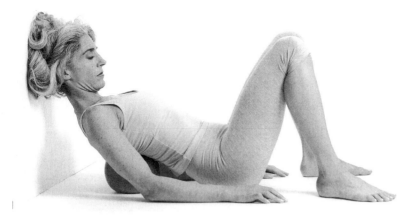

Step 4

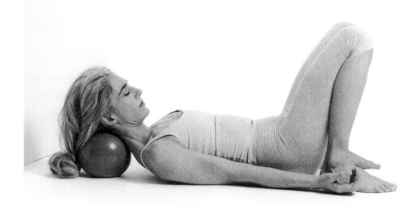

Step 6

4. Continue to roll the ball up the right side of your spine, pausing at each vertebra, just as in the basic back routine (pages 60–68), only keeping your back, head, and neck against the wall.

5. By the time the ball is at your shoulder blades, you will begin to come away from the wall. From this point on your head will not be resting on the wall, so you must use your left hand to support your head by pulling your chin toward your chest to keep the back of your neck long.

6. Continue rolling up the rest of your spine as in the regular back routine, steps 9 to 13 (pages 190–94).

7. Repeat on the left side.

Chair Routines

Anyone confined to a chair can do the chair routines described in chapters 4 and 6:

- Back Routine, pages 75–76. If you don't have the flexibility to move the ball behind your back on your own, you may need a helper or caregiver to move it for you.

- Leg Routines: for the hamstrings (pages 118–19), quadriceps (page 120), and inner thighs (page 121). Again, you may need some assistance.

Foot Routines in a Chair

No matter what your age, it's important to keep your feet healthy, toned, and flexible. You can do both variations of the foot routine in a seated position, which makes them less intense for sensitive feet. If you want to put more pressure on your feet, lean your weight forward and rest your forearms on top of your legs.

This way of working your feet won't create as much of a muscle release as standing on the balls (see pages 131–37), but you will get a gentle stimulation of the bones and muscles of the feet that prevents fluid buildup and increases circulation.

Use a solid rubber ball (called a sponge ball) about two and a half inches in diameter. It should be firm, not soft. As instructed previously, don't use a golf ball or Superball—they're much too hard *and will injure you.* Don't use a tennis ball or any other hollow ball, for it will indent when you put weight into it, rather than giving like solid

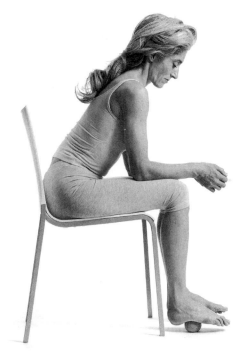

Foot routine in chair

rubber. The best ball I have found is the Pinky, which is widely available at drugstores and chain stores such as Kmart and Wal-Mart. You will need two balls so you can work both feet together.

VARIATION 1

This simpler version of the foot routine is good to start out with. These instructions apply to both feet at the same time.

1. While sitting in a chair, place the ball under the center of your heel, with your foot pointing straight in front of you. Stay like this for 15 to 30 seconds.

2. Microshift, bringing your leg slightly backward so the ball rolls just off your heel into the beginning of your arch. Part of the

ball still touches the heel. You're moving the ball toward your toes, right through the center line of the foot. Let the weight of the leg sink into the ball. Hold for 15 to 30 seconds.

Tip for step 2

- *It's very important here to keep your arches lifted and your feet pointing straight ahead.*

3. Microshift so the ball rolls a bit farther into the arch and hold as in step 2.

4. Continue to roll down the arch, holding at each point, until your weight distribution changes and your heel has to come down to the floor. At this point the ball will be just at the beginning of the ball of the foot, still on the center line.

Tip for step 4

- *The ball of the foot is the padding that makes up the widest part of the foot, just beneath the toes; it extends across the entire foot, from the big toe to the pinky.*

5. Continue working the ball up over the ball of the foot, toward the toes. Stay at each point for 15 to 30 seconds.

6. Continue rolling in small increments until the ball has reached the beginning of your toes and you can spread your toes out over the ball and grip it. Lean your weight into the ball and stay like this for 15 to 30 seconds.

7. Slide the ball out until it reaches the tips of your toes. The ball of the foot is almost on the floor and the toes are stretched out over the ball. Stay here for 15 to 30 seconds.

Tips for step 7

- *Unlike step 6, you're not gripping the ball here; you're letting it stretch your toes long.*

- *If the ball pops out from under your toes, do this step against a piece of furniture or a book braced against a wall.*

8. Take both balls away and check for any differences in the way your feet feel.

VARIATION 2

Once you've become used to working the feet with Variation 1, try this variation, which works the sides of the foot separately from the center and will more effectively tone and lift your arches.

1. Follow steps 1 to 5 in Variation 1, except that at each point, after holding for 15 to 30 seconds, move the ball from the center to the outside of the foot. Hold again, then move the ball to the inside edge of the foot and hold. Then bring the ball back to center and roll to the next point. Continue working down the foot this way until both heels are resting on the floor.

Tips for step 1

- *Always move to the outside of the foot first. Working the outside edge raises the arch, making it less painful to press the ball under the inside edge.*

- *Make sure you keep your ankles from turning inward; it's very easy to lose your alignment during this routine. To correct inward-turning ankles, instead of trying to keep your knees straight in front of you, turn them outward. This will keep your ankles from dropping.*

2. When the ball reaches the beginning of the toes, grip it with the three center toes and hold for 15 to 30 seconds (as in step 6 of Variation 1). Then move it to the outside edge and grip with the last three toes. Finally, move it to the inside edge and grip it with the big toe and second toe.

3. When the ball of the foot comes down to the floor (corresponding to step 7 in Variation 1), stretch the three central toes over the ball, then the outside three toes, and finally the big toe and second toe, holding for 15 to 30 seconds each time.

Shoulder Release

You can use the frozen shoulder routine on pages 181–82 to keep your shoulders from getting stiff. By wedging the ball into the armpit, you separate the bones and muscles of the shoulder, making the joint more flexible. It's a great way to open the shoulder, release the neck, and increase the oxygen supply into the chest, shoulder, and head. You can do this routine either standing or sitting in a chair.

Bed Routines

People confined to bed can easily develop problems with blood circulation, as well as muscle atrophy. Rolling down the backs of the legs and up the spine is wonderful for keeping the blood moving and muscles toned and to reduce the chance of developing bedsores.

Most people in bed will need a helper to actually roll the ball. The helper should use only as much pressure as feels comfortable for you. The pressure should feel pleasant and relaxing, not painful or uncomfortable.

For these routines you should use a soft ball about six inches in diameter. In the leg or neck routines, where you don't feel the expansion of the torso against the ball, use your breath to pace your movement by taking a full breath at each point, as described on page 53. The caregiver can watch your rib cage and abdomen expand and contract as a cue for when to move the ball.

Back Routine in Bed

There are several ways for a person in bed to do the back routine. Be sure you roll the ball along either side of the spine, *not* in the center.

- If you can move around in bed, try lying on the ball and rolling up each side of the spine by yourself.

- If you need assistance, lie on your back. Have your helper gently lift your pelvis and scoot the ball underneath your sacrum. The ball will sink into the bed, so there won't be a lot of strain on your lower back. The helper then moves the ball up your back in small increments, reminding you to take one full breath at each point. If it's comfortable, the helper can roll all the way to the top of your head on both sides.

- If you can lie facedown, the helper can gently roll the ball up from the sacrum in small increments, using very light pressure. At each point the helper should pause, so you can breathe and feel your back expanding against the ball. Roll as far up the neck as possible.

Leg Routines in Bed

My active older clients often do these routines in the morning before getting out of bed in order to warm up their hamstrings and prevent morning stiffness. For bedridden people, these routines are great for stimulating circulation and keeping the muscles toned.

Hamstring Release in Bed

1. Lie on your back. Lift your right leg (or have someone do it for you) and place the ball up against your right sitbone (for instructions on finding your sitbone, see page 49).

Tip for step 1

- *Since the ball sinks into the bed, the right hip will be only slightly elevated. As the ball moves down the leg, both hips will rest flat on the bed.*

2. Lower your right leg to rest on the ball and remain for 15 to 20 seconds, breathing and feeling the leg sink into the ball.

Tip for step 2

- *Since the response time of a person in bed will be longer, the pauses for waiting and sinking must be longer as well, to let the stimulation and release occur.*

3. Raise your leg, roll the ball down a little farther, and lower the leg over the ball again. Wait and breathe as before.

4. Continue rolling the ball, in small increments, all the way to the ankle. If you can, use your left foot to push the right leg down against the ball.

5. Repeat on the left side.

Quadriceps Routine in Bed

Doing this quadriceps routine on the bed will elongate and stimulate these muscles without the same intense sensation you might experience when doing the routine on the floor, since the bed has more give.

1. Lie on your right side. Place the ball at the top of your right thigh, then roll onto your stomach so your leg rests on the ball. Hold it here for 10 seconds. Your left leg should be extended behind you on the bed, and you can use it to help you balance on the ball. Rest your head on your folded arms in front of you, or, if you need extra help balancing, bend your arms so your

forearms rest on the bed with your fingertips at the level of your shoulders.

2. With your right hand, push the ball down the right leg in small increments, holding for 10 seconds at each point, until the ball is just above the knee.

3. If you can't lie facedown, a helper can roll the ball down your thigh, pressing gently (as much as is comfortable). Hold for 10 seconds at each point.

4. Repeat on the left side.

Inner Thigh Routine on Your Back

Active people can use this and the next routine to strengthen, stretch, and tone the adductor muscles. When you stand up afterward, you'll feel well balanced and stable, with your legs solidly supporting your torso.

1. Lie on your back and separate your legs slightly. Place the ball between your legs, as close to the pubic bone as possible. Squeeze your legs together around the ball and hold for 5 to 10 seconds.

2. Continue moving the ball down your thighs, squeezing your legs together and holding for 5 to 10 seconds at each point, until you reach your knees.

Inner Thigh Routine on Your Front

Do this routine if you can lie facedown with one knee bent out to the side.

1. Lying facedown, bend your right knee out to the side at hip level.

2. Place the ball underneath you at the inner groin of the bent leg and rest, cradling your head in your arms.

3. Slowly move your body to the left so the ball rolls out toward the right knee. Continue rolling the ball out toward the knee, an inch at a time, holding for 10 seconds at each point.

4. Repeat on the left side.

Resources

To get rolling right now, visit the Yamuna® Body Rolling website, www.yamunabodyrolling.com, where you'll find everything you need:

- The specially designed Yamuna® Body Rolling balls and Foot Savers

- A small, easily packable pump that you can take with you to deflate and reinflate your ball while traveling

- The six Yamuna® Body Rolling videos, which range from 10 to 60 minutes in length and cover everything from a full-body workout to a brief session for the office

- Other Yamuna® Body Rolling products

- A list of certified Yamuna® Body Rolling practitioners all over the United States, as well as in Canada, England, Italy, Spain, Argentina, Israel, Singapore, and Hong Kong

- A schedule of Yamuna® Body Rolling classes taught at my studio in New York and by certified practitioners elsewhere

- Information about Yamuna® Body Rolling certification training

You can also call 1–888–226–9616 or 1–800–877–8429 to order Yamuna® Body Rolling products, request our product catalog, or find certified practitioners in your area. All Yamuna® Body Rolling products can be purchased from your local practitioner.